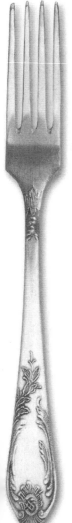
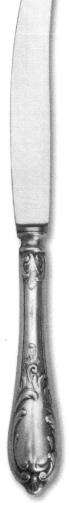

STUFFED

how to feel so good about yourself you won't have room for cake

Fadela Hilali

PRAISE

'If you are an Emotional Eater, you need to read this book. It's that simple. Fadela doesn't sugar coat anything – she keeps it real and tells it like it is. Plus, she backs it all up with proper scientific facts in an easy to read way. She is completely open about her own struggles to help you overcome your own. And of course it wouldn't be Fadela's book without her honesty, understanding and humour. This awesome book should be the go-to for Emotional Eating help!'

Michael Serwa, High-end Life Coach,
Speaker and Author of *From Good to Amazing*

'Fadela Hilali's book, *Stuffed*, is insightful and a pleasure to read. I'm sure it will be a great source of support for its readers. Fadela writes in a style that makes the material accessible and relevant. It feels like having a conversation with a trusted friend. She interweaves life lessons and scientific research in order to offer help and advice to anyone who suffers with emotional eating. If you recognise that in yourself and you want to change your relationship with food, *Stuffed* can provide you with the tools to help you do it.'

Dr Amani Zarroug, Clinical Psychologist

'Finally a book that explains why eating can feel so out of control. Fadela shares her journey with so much honesty, highlighting the triggers and stories that so many of us can relate to. Had I had a book like this 20 years ago, I would have been a happier woman appreciating my beauty inside out and most probably enjoying my food all the way. If you want to get to the bottom of your unhealthy relationship or obsession with food (or no food) once and for all, this book is a must-read.'

Duda Jadrijevic, Buddhist Coach, Speaker & Serial Entrepreneur
www.kickassmuse.com

'An amazing read. Incredibly well researched with a plethora of scientific backup, along with Fadela's own experiences. All this said, it is a very light read (over a heavy topic), Fadela's humour really comes out here and makes it an absolute pleasure to read. There are many lessons to learn about emotional eating, our psychology, our limiting beliefs and what is behind it all with some great practical tips to help everyone enjoy food the way it should be enjoyed and how to love ourselves more. I've learned so much from this amazingly written book and had a good laugh too. It's the equivalent of that teacher you loved at school who made learning easy, effective and fun, whose class you couldn't wait for (and I very seldom went to class so this means a lot!).'

Alexander Tadj-Saadat, Life Coach and Speaker

'Fadela shares her own story from the beginning and sets the tone for a book that isn't about preaching, but rather about understanding and guidance. This book is easy to read, yet jam-packed with key insights. *Stuffed* goes way beneath the surface of emotional eating to get right down to the nitty-gritty at the heart of the problem. There's no fooling Fadela, or yourself, with this book, she knows and exposes all the secrets and proves you are far from being alone in this spiral. Take her hand, turn the page and take charge of your habits for a happier, healthier life all round.'

Thandi Demanet, Senior Conference Producer

R**ETHINK** PRESS

First published in Great Britain 2017
by Rethink Press (www.rethinkpress.com)

© Copyright Fadela Hilali

Cover image © Volodymyr Krasyuk / Shutterstock

CONTENTS

To my mother, a living example of unconditional love, determination and resilience.

INTRODUCTION

I wonder why we're here. My mum said it was an important meeting and the man opening the door looks very serious… and round. He welcomes us, shakes my hand and walks us to his desk. Who is this guy? I look around for clues and notice the frames hanging on the wall behind him. His name is Dr A and he is a dietician. He seems out of breath. He reminds me of Mr Greedy from the Mister Men books. I chuckle; my mum shoots me a look. Oh wait, he is talking to me now. 'Hello Fadela.' I flash my teeth in a smile, I hope I'm not in trouble. He continues, 'You are a big girl now, and I'm sure you will understand what I'm going to tell you.' Awkward silence. 'If you keep on eating the way you do, you will be very fat and unhappy. Do you understand?' I nod. He continues talking but my mind is wandering and I only catch fragments of the conversation he is now having with my mum: 'Drink water before she eats', 'no bread or pasta'. He is scribbling on a white pad and my mum is also taking notes. I'm bored. Oh, he is talking to me again: 'Fadela, just remember,' he says, 'the pleasure of eating lasts a moment, but fat will stay with you forever.' I nod again and look at the clock behind him. It's almost time for my basketball practice. I don't want to be late.

This meeting was my first encounter with a dietician. I was eight years old and my parents were concerned that their divorce had caused my recent weight gain and a habit of seeking comfort in food. They looked for an expert and Dr A turned out to be the only dietician in my home town. Dr A was also obese, morbidly obese. Instead of reassuring my parents that I needed some time to adjust and emotional reassurance that we were still OK as a family, or maybe a few lifestyle tweaks, Dr A gave me a strict diet. I hated everything about it and quit it after just a week. This was to be the first of *many* diets I would struggle with throughout my life.

Parents' divorce aside, I was a happy kid and I have fond memories of my childhood. I was the youngest of three sisters and because there was such a big age gap between us (my eldest sister Narmine is fifteen years older than me and my sister Asmaa is seven years older) I was smothered with attention. I was given all the free passes I could dream of and if there was ever a dispute between us, our mum would gently remind them that I was the youngest and that they should cut me some slack. That, they did. My every need was catered to. I got everything I wanted. I didn't have to compete with anyone for attention. I was loved.

Many of my childhood memories revolve around play, school trips, and family gatherings but I also have vivid food recollections. I can trace back my earliest memory of food to when I was five. We were staying in our family home in Rabat, Morocco. My parents were out and I was taking full advantage of it by playing with all the electronics usually off-limits. Within minutes of getting my grubby little hands on the TV remote, I dropped it and it looked broken. Panic. My five-year-old self came up with an immediate solution: 'You must hide until they're not mad at you so take enough provisions for a couple of days.' I ran to the kitchen, grabbed a bag of Haribo sweets, made my way to one of the bedrooms upstairs and hid behind a big armchair. I felt prepared. These sweets could last me for a couple of days, or so I thought. The sweets must have lasted an hour at which point I realised that my plan had some fundamental flaws. So I made my way out of my hiding place, repentant and ready to confess. Many years later, Haribo sweets were still my go-to emergency food.

I never became obese (the morbidly obese nutritionist gets no credit for that!) but that first diet did nothing but exacerbate my overeating. I knew I was overweight, the kids in school made sure I was aware of that. I knew I liked to eat when I was sad or upset, but I'd never felt out of control around food, not until I experimented with restricting food. My relationship with food was never the same after my first diet. From there on, food was either fattening or slimming. I started to feel guilty about eating sweets and the guiltier I felt, the more sweets I ate. I would try to undo the perceived damage by restricting my food intake for a day or two. I would get *so* much encouragement from everyone around me whenever I lost weight: 'You've lost weight, look at how pretty you are'; or the alternative, disapproving looks at the sight of my big thighs accompanied by: 'You've gained weight sweetie, it's such a shame'.

That first diet was followed by many more which included Herbal Life, the 7 Day Cabbage Soup, Weight Watchers, Atkins, Detoxes, High Protein diets, Meat diets, Slim Fast and a few more from random magazines and the internet… You name it, I've probably tried it! Unsurprisingly, I ended up developing an eating disorder and depression by the time I was 15. It started with anorexia, followed by bulimia and binge eating. After a few years of struggle, I did eventually heal from my eating disorder phase but I went straight back to alternating between emotional eating and the yo-yo dieting I was oh-so-familiar with. My self-love was still close to nil and my quest for the perfect body that would give me the perfect life was ongoing. At the end of my second year in university in Charleston, I decided to invest my meagre savings in a personal trainer. The tips he gave me were sensible and I did try really hard to follow his advice, but only sometimes. By then it was becoming clear to me that willpower was not my issue and I had plenty of evidence in different areas of my life to back it up. The measurement days were invariably the same. I would look down sheepishly repeating that I didn't understand why I made no progress. I only indulged in a vanilla latte once in a while, that's it, and maybe a smoothie after the gym. I completely believed the words that came out of my mouth. I was in total denial.

I knew everything there was to know about nutrition. I was a calorie expert, an exercise bunny, and a pretty emotionally aware human being thanks to years of therapy. But awareness and knowledge were not enough to make me put the spoon down when I was full or walk away from the sweet aisle in a supermarket. Nothing came even close to the comfort I found staying alone in my bedroom, watching my favourite TV shows and eating; eating myself numb. Food always delivered. Boy doesn't call back? Ice cream. Bad grade? Chocolate. Argument with family? Fast food. Hangover? Indian buffet. I no longer had an eating disorder per se but I was still hooked to emotional eating.

I also had good days where food was just food and I felt on top of my emotions, completely in charge of my life. My love for exercise played a huge role in those days. Maybe because my mum used to leave a Jane Fonda exercise tape playing to distract me as a toddler when she was leaving for work, or maybe because I find it so easy to make friends at the gym. Either way, exercising indubitably helped me claw myself out of depression.

My first emotional breakthrough came in 2006 after a semester abroad in Trujillo, Spain. I was working with Dr Zazzaro at the time, a brilliant therapist based in Charleston. We were focusing on my self-esteem and unhealthy relationship with food and whilst I was making great progress with my self-awareness, food was still an issue.

Trujillo is a beautiful medieval town where a 13th-century castle proudly stands. The rhythm of life is slower there and people seem mellow. I couldn't help but notice how the locals enjoyed their food. It was convivial and meals lasted for hours sometimes. I loved my time there, everything about it felt right. This isn't to say that life was perfect or easy, it wasn't. Most of the girls in our small group were part of a sorority and I didn't particularly fit in. I lived with a traditional Spanish family with three generations under the same roof and very little privacy. But it didn't matter, I felt good. Not elated, not overly excited, just good. I ate whatever the family was eating (Spanish food is not diet-friendly), made local friends and surprise, surprise, lost weight. I lost weight without dieting, without having access to any fat-free or sugar-free food. No gym membership either; I walked every day to my classes (right by the castle), I swam a bit, exercised in the garden whenever I felt like it and it felt right.

It was also so refreshing to see people so relaxed about their body. Older and younger women alike pampered themselves before meeting their friends for a drink in the Plaza in the evening. They didn't seem to care about loose flesh and cellulite or if they did, it certainly didn't stop them from wearing what they liked. I, on the other hand, still didn't own a single pair of shorts because of how self-conscious I was about my legs.

Whilst the local lifestyle wasn't necessarily something my restless, 100-miles per hour, ambitious mind aspired to, it was the first time in years I wasn't worried about my future, what people thought, what they expected, or who I wanted to be. I completely adapted to their lifestyle and went with the flow. I was present, playful and, dare I say it, happy. I was Stuffed. My mum visited me in Spain and she too was completely blown away by how happy I was. We both naively thought that the Spanish lifestyle had succeeded in teaching me self-love where everything else had failed before.

After eight weeks of Spanish bliss, I went back to sunny Charleston in South Carolina glowing, ten pounds lighter and with a renewed sense of joy at the life I could finally have. The post-Spain high lasted an entire academic year. I felt on top of the world. Food was, well, just food. Exercise was still my friend and the extreme mood swings were gone! It was one of my best years. I was doing great in my studies, working part-time, and had a great group of friends. I also made the decision to move to Spain for my Master's degree. It's around that time that my gremlins resurfaced. Was I making the right decision? Was I ready to move to Spain? Was I ready for postgraduate studies? Was I really leaving *everything* I knew behind? The doubt was excruciating so I turned to my most trusted friend: food.

The years following university followed a similar pattern. I would get the job I wanted and feel on top of the world for a while but the excitement would wear off and the uncomfortable emotions would re-emerge. As I approached my mid-twenties, it became quite clear that I was trapped. I was trapped by my desperate attempts to stop feeling. I was trapped in my deeply ingrained dysfunctional habits. Always worrying about food and gaining weight is tiring. I was tired, so tired. I knew by that time that when I felt good, overeating or eating for the sake of it did not appeal to me at all. Where I tried to tackle food as the root of my problems in the past, I was now looking at food as a symptom of my emotional discomfort. It seems so obvious today and yet, it was a complete game changer, a game changer that would spark a phase of experimentation that led me to bolster my emotional resilience. I felt good in my own skin. I also developed new strategies to help me deal with my emotions and none of them involved the use of food. That's when I started feeling Stuffed.

My journey to feeling good was very intuitive and full of trial and error. I also did a lot of research, research that helped me understand why my diets always failed and why my relationship with food had been so dysfunctional. I'm the kind of (annoying) person who needs to understand everything. Having scientific evidence to back up my own painful conclusions about dieting, bingeing and disordered eating was empowering. All those years I wished I could eat like everyone else – you know, be normal around food – but it turned out I was far from being alone.

This book is what I would have wanted to gift to myself when I was feeling so helpless, battling food with no end in sight. This book is about finding emotional freedom and never sending another one of us to a battle we can't win. Leave no one behind. The war is over and it's time to feel Stuffed.

Part One

WHY YOU ARE NOT STUFFED –
WHAT GOT YOU HERE

Whether you have a history of disordered eating, whether you actually need to lose weight or not, whether you've yo-yo dieted yourself through adulthood, the reason you turn to food is not from a lack of information. As a modern society, we are obsessed with looks – slim looks, to be more accurate. Diets are everywhere and young children are under increasing pressure to keep up with what they see on social media.

In the last five years, our obsession with food has reached new heights. Paleo, Vegan, Raw Vegan, Sugar-Free, Gluten-Free, Dairy-Free, Alkaline, Plant-based, Grain-free, Mediterranean, Juice Fasting, Clean Eating, and many more trends I'm probably unaware of are flooding social media. A few still advertise traditional diets but many have opted for the Clean Eating trend. Everyone is posting about their food, desperately trying to find their place within an oh-so-complicated food spectrum. We're experiencing the rise of food indoctrination, as if we couldn't trust ourselves (and our body) to figure out the fuel we need.

What we eat is now everyone's business, out in the open. We have so little faith in our natural ability to keep ourselves healthy that we are willing to believe anything and anyone dishing us a healthy lifestyle with a side of unhealthy body perfectionism. Some people live by these trends and feel great about it. Good for them. My guess is that if you are reading this book, a part of you is still looking for answers. You can eat clean on Instagram and still binge on weekends. You can eat paleo during the day and pig out on your kids' snacks in the evening. You can eat clean and have *no* energy and feel awful because your body is not getting what it needs from the picture perfect food you're giving it.

Even when I was still deep in my emotional eating, people around me thought I was as healthy as they come. All they ever saw me eat was unprocessed food, fruit and salads. I was eating healthy in public, supposedly completely over dieting, but food was still my dirty little secret. Beyond that, my obsession with 'healthy' food had an awful lot in common with my attitude towards food when I had an eating disorder. I now know that this has a name too, it's called orthorexia. Orthorexia is about eating correctly or the obsession with eating healthy food where one systematically avoids specific foods they believe to be unhealthy. Thinking back to my behaviour in those days, I fit that description to a T.

There are numerous health gurus on today's scene and many of them promote plant-based eating. I am not here to judge or demonise anyone but what I will say is that I have seen some rather preposterous pseudo-scientific claims such as people recommending eating nothing but potatoes for an entire year. As you now know, my first experience with a dietician wasn't great but there are thankfully plenty of good dieticians in the world. It is also worth mentioning that dieticians are regulated in the UK, nutritionists aren't. Many of today's health gurus have disclaimers on their websites clearly stating that while their food philosophy is free from wheat, dairy, meat and refined sugar (I need to catch my breath here), they emphasise that it's a personal decision. Fair is fair. They share tips based on their own experience with food and their body and that is fine by me. But let me ask you this: if they found the right balance for them through trial and error, based on their own body characteristics and medical history, what's preventing the rest of us from doing the same? I'm not here to demonise anybody. I follow lots of wellness and food accounts on social media because, frankly, I love how pretty the pictures look. While I may not want to make my eating exclusively plant-based, I love getting inspiration for new recipes, but instead of making a salad my main meal, I might decide to make it a side. There is nothing wrong with eating more vegetable and fruit. On the contrary, the point here is to realise that regardless of the latest wellness trend, I know what I need to feel good. I know what my ideal health blueprint is, both mental and physical. And so can you. But don't worry, you need not do this alone. I am right here with you.

Let's begin.

Why you can't stick to a diet

As much as we don't like to admit it, we know deep down that dieting is a never-ending cycle. We know that losing weight gets harder and harder each time and that while our dieting rules become more extreme, the results are much harder to achieve. It's depressing and sometimes we wish we could forget about it all and just enjoy life. So we do, but because we've been on a cycle of deprivation for so long, we don't even know what it's like to enjoy a 'normal' life. So we go for all the 'forbidden' food – things we've come to label 'naughty' – but we deserve it, right? We've been *so* good; it's all about balance, they say. And at first it feels good. We thoroughly enjoy eating out without worrying about the healthy options available on the menu; we feel full and we still order dessert because, well, we might as well go all out. But slowly reality creeps back in, along with a sugar crash, lethargy and, of course, guilt. The guilt train is never late.

How could you do that? You've undone all the hard work you did. You feel huge; you feel disgusted with yourself. The mean voice in your head goes wild. Mine sounded like this: 'You're worthless! You're weak, gross, and a waste of space! No one will ever love you, you don't deserve to be loved.' And because I'd been through it before, more times than I wished to remember, I knew exactly what to do next. So I made myself (and the mean voice) a promise, the same promise I always made after going off the rails. I'll get back on track on Monday. I'll be so good, no more over-indulging or bingeing. I will stick to the plan: healthy food all the way. It's the new me. I will be healthy. I'll be *so* good! No, seriously, this time I mean it!

And I would genuinely believe this promise and try my best to honour it. But then something would go wrong, the way things always go wrong in life. I would get into a fight with my boyfriend, or my boss would decide to turn into a giant pain or I simply felt so tired, stressed and drained. I would make my way home feeling low and my thoughts would turn to food, the way we turn to a good friend for comfort. Cupboards and fridge inventory done, trip to the supermarket if the food available wasn't 'low mood' friendly, I would go for it, oblivious. Oblivious to the consequences of breaking the healthy slim promise I made myself, time and time again. It felt good, it always did, in an almost numbing kind of way... until my consciousness resurfaced. I would take in the empty wrappers around me, the empty tub of ice cream, the half-finished box of cookies, the discomfort in my belly. In a matter of seconds horror would wash over me. *What did I do?*

Horrified by my lack of willpower, I would vow to work out the next day. I would eat healthily or I wouldn't eat to make up for it! I would swear I'd be stronger next time. I'd be good, for good… until it happened again. And it always did. This is what I've now come to describe as the **dieting cycle of helplessness**.

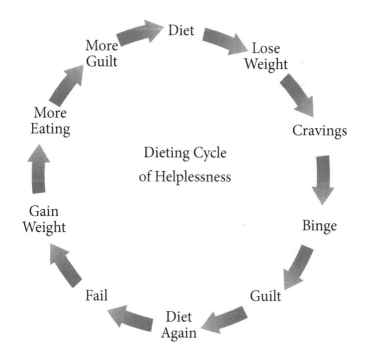

We all deserve better than to be at war with food and our body. I know what it's like to be stuck in that cycle of helplessness. I also know that it's hard to admit that controlling food is not the answer. If a part of you is not

17

entirely convinced that there is no diet that will fix how you feel about food, that's fine because that's the story we've been told. But that story hasn't served you or me, so how about rewriting it once and for all? This chapter will look at some of the main reasons diets seldom work. You may find yourself thinking, 'Come on, it can be that bad!' It is; it's *that* bad. The weight loss industry is worth over two billion dollars in the United States (US) alone, that's how bad it is. My personal struggles as well as my experience working with my private coaching clients with a dieting history gives me valuable insights on the matter, but I assure you that the information you are about to read is all drawn from referenced scientific sources.

Research is now all but unanimous that diets do not lead to sustainable weight loss for the majority of people. Not only that, but most dieters gain weight after coming off a diet and end up heavier than when they started.

One of the first things dieters notice is an increase in food cravings. Our human psychology is pretty simple on that point – the more scarce something is, the more we want it. Think of all the limited editions that make us go out of our way to buy them: the collectable Coca-Cola bottle or a limited edition MAC lipstick. We are told to completely ban certain food groups from our mind, heart and kitchen. The problem with trying to stop thinking about something is that you are, ironically, still thinking about it. If I asked you not to think about a pink elephant, chances are you would find it extremely hard to get the image of a pink elephant out of your head. The obsession with food combined with the scarcity of it makes for a potent combination.

There is an underlying assumption that women are the prime candidates for diets and that the war against food is a female prerogative but it does also affect men. As a matter of fact, one of the most famous dieting studies in the history of nutrition highlighting the impact of calorie restrictions was conducted on male participants.

In 1944, 36 young, healthy, psychologically fit young men volunteered to participate in a study of human semi-starvation conducted by professor Ancel Keys and some of his colleagues from the University of Minnesota.[a] The study, eventually known as the Minnesota Starvation Experiment, was designed to learn about the physical and psychological effects of partial starvation experienced by civilians during World War II. This study was commissioned by the US War Department and is still instrumental in the scientific study of nutrition.

---

[a] Leah M. Kalm *et al.* 'They Starved So That Others Be Better Fed: Remembering Ancel Keys and the Minnesota Experiment.' *The Journal of Nutrition* (2005)

The study was divided into three different phases: observation under normal eating conditions for three months (3200 kcal), observation during a semi-starvation phase for six months (1800 kcal), and observation throughout the 'refeeding' rehabilitation phase for a further three months.

The participants were all keen to be a part of the study, but their enthusiasm quickly faded as the semi-starvation phase progressed. In addition to physical symptoms like tiredness, dizziness and weakness, they also became more irritable. Does this sound familiar? It goes on – food became an obsession, with one participant recalling how it wasn't so much about actual hunger but about food becoming the most important thing in life. Participants also reported a lack of interest in dating and a complete lack of sex drive.

On average, the participants lost 25% of their body weight throughout the study. Two participants were excluded from the study during the semi-starvation phase for not adhering to the calories allowed. The men in question reported more disturbing behaviours like stopping at different shops to buy sundaes, stealing food, scavenging through bins and chewing up to 40 packs of gum a day! The participants' psychological distress eventually led to brief stays in psychiatric wards too. It's worth reiterating that all men were assessed before the study and deemed psychologically healthy.

Other observations of participants drawn from the semi-starvation part of the study included new obsessions in food, collecting hundreds of new cookbooks, compulsive food planning, increased self-criticism, loss of muscle mass, anxiety, mood swings and isolation.

As the participants started preparing to move on to their rehabilitation period, they were told to slowly ease back into a normal diet and to be careful not to go all out. The advice was acknowledged, but they still felt out of control. One participant ate so much that he ended up getting his stomach pumped; another one ate several meals (and vomited on a bus afterwards) because he 'couldn't satisfy [his] craving for food by filling up [his] stomach.' The rehabilitation period also came with frequent feelings of guilt and shame followed by out-of-control eating episodes, known as binges, which we will look at in more detail.

So when you think back to the last time you flunked your diet and ate an entire tray of cookies, you can know with absolute certainty that you are not the problem.

Cravings

A craving can be defined as 'an intense desire to consume a particular food (or type of food) that is difficult to resist'.[b] The main difference between a food craving and normal hunger is that hunger can be satisfied by eating any type of food while a craving will only be alleviated with a particular kind of food.[c] If you've ever been on a diet, you will have noticed that you start craving the foods that you've restricted within a couple of days of dieting, or sometimes before you even start. Let's be honest, our body's optimal functioning does not *need* Ben and Jerry's peanut butter ice cream or a cheese-stuffed-crust pepperoni pizza.

Interestingly, scientists have found when studying the brains of smokers, alcoholics and overeaters that the structure of their brain (neurology) changes as their cravings increase in frequency. Very strong habits have the same effects as addictions in that the desire for something, like food, can turn into obsessive thoughts leading us to act on the craving on autopilot. This impulse behaviour will occur regardless of the negative consequences it will yield. We know that excessive eating will feel uncomfortable afterwards and, if done

---

[b] White, Marney A. *et al.* 'Development and Validation of the Food-Craving Inventory.' Obesity Research (2002)
[c] Pelchat, Marcia Levin *et al.* 'Dietary Monotony and Food Cravings in Young and Elderly Adults.' Physiology & Behavior (2000)

consistently, lead to weight gain, but it's not enough to stop us from doing it.[d.]

When we learn to anticipate eating chocolate whenever we are sad or stressed we, often unconsciously, develop a habit that strengthens over time. We learn that eating chocolate, or another type of food, soothes us. When we are sad or stressed, but don't get the 'fix' we anticipated, we end up with an unfulfilled craving that leads to frustration.[e.] This is particularly true for very tasty foods, known as palatable foods. The effect of the palatable foods we tend to consume when emotionally eating is reinforced through the activation of the reward pathways in our brain, the same process occurring in the brain of individuals with drug and alcohol addictions.

Binge eating

Binge eating is the act of consuming excessive food that is *not* driven by hunger. It typically involves eating large quantities that lead to uncomfortable fullness. Binge eating episodes habitually come with feelings of powerlessness, guilt and emotional distress.

[d.] Charles Duhigg *The Power of Habit: Why We Do What We Do in Life and Business* (2012)
[e.] Ibid

Drawing from my own experience and that of the clients I have worked with, the food chosen for a binge, or a 'feast' as some like to call it, usually involves calorie rich foods that are banned from most diets. Some of my previously forbidden foods included cake, pasta, pizza, chocolate, sweets, and ice cream. And when I mean forbidden, I would not even allow myself to be near them. OK, most days of the week, except for Friday night… and Saturday evening… and Sunday.

Several of my friends in the fitness industry also relate to these patterns. I was really curious to find out if personal trainers experienced similar challenges with their clients' body transformations so I asked one of my Personal Trainer friends, let's call him Alan. We didn't get a chance to talk about his clients because Alan went off on a tangent about his own challenges before and after bodybuilding competitions.

If you are not familiar with the bodybuilding world, there are two different phases that athletes go through. The first one is known as 'bulking' and consists of eating excess calories and training to build up muscle. The next phase is all about 'cutting', the dieting period leading to up to a competition which requires cutting calories and carbs to lose fat and get as lean as possible for the big day. Alan told me that while he loved winning these competitions, the journey was emotionally draining, especially during the 'cutting' phase. All he could think about was food. A loaf of bread inadvertently left in plain sight by his girlfriend felt like torture. He would go to a coffee shop and buy chocolate brownies, six or seven of them. He would sit at a table and look at them for a while before giving them away. He showed me a picture of him when he won the Miami Pro World Championship and a picture of him three days later on holiday with his girlfriend. It was hard to believe how much he'd increased in size! There was some water retention but he also said that all he did for three days was eat and eat and eat until he couldn't move. He jokingly calls it a food coma. As uncomfortable as this may sound, Alan puts himself through the same process once or twice a year to compete at the level he's at and he is far from being alone. Try typing 'binge eating bodybuilding' in your Internet browser and you will get a sense of the scope of the problem.

So there you have it, there are no exceptions. No one is immune to bingeing. Whether you are a bodybuilder, a model, or an emotional eater, research clearly shows that restricting food intake and dieting increase the chances of binge eating.

Overeating

Overeating is a less extreme form of dysfunctional eating, but an important one nonetheless when looking at emotional eating and causes of weight gain. In a study, researchers studying the link between dieting and binge eating found that 'psychological deprivation, induced by short periods of caloric restriction, is enough to trigger overeating and increase hunger.'[f] The 2009 study was conducted on a group of young, healthy individuals who were put on a four-week diet where they consumed 600 calories per day four days per week and ate as much as they wanted the rest of the week. This is actually the premise of the 5:2 diet or intermittent fasting that became so popular in 2013. The researchers found that the participants substantially increased the calories they consumed on the days they could eat as much as they wanted compared to what they used to eat before participating in the study (baseline). Side effects of restricting their calorie intake four days of the week included irritability, fatigue, low mood, poor concentration and, wait for it, no significant weight loss. This is a trend that has been observed in other studies where it has also been suggested that compulsive dieters do not lose weight over time, regardless of how often they try.[g] According to Dr Sandra Aamot, dieting tends to make people more overweight because it affects their natural ability to recognise hunger which, in turn, makes them more likely to eat emotionally.[h]

---

[f] Randi E. McCabe, 'Exposing the Diet Myth: Diets Make You Eat Less' (1999)
[g] Ibid
[h] Sandra Aamot, *Why Diets Make Us Fat* (2016)

There is another common phenomenon among people with a history of restricting food and/or dieting known as 'Too late now' or 'Screw it'. This happens when we fall off whatever 'eating plan' we were following and decide that we might as well go all out... until Monday. In an emotional eater and dieter's mind, Monday is the equivalent of a new year's resolution, but one with an even shorter life span.

Mood swings

Mood swings, irritability, negative thoughts and sadness are all regularly experienced by dieters. Studies have now shown that poor eating behaviours, including bingeing, overeating and unhealthy eating, can negatively impact our mood.

Kristin Heron, a research associate at Penn State University explains that while there were no noticeable changes in her research participants' mood before a disordered eating episode, there was a clear dip in their mood afterwards.[i] Another study suggests that there may be a link between overindulging on junk foods and the occurrence of depression and depression-like behaviour.[j]

---

[i] Nauert, Rick. Poor eating behaviors can worsen mood | Psych central news. 2013
[j] Sànchez-Villegas, A. *et al.*'Fast-food and commercial baked goods consumption and the risk of depression' (2012)

Deborah Colson, a specialist in nutritional support for mental health and neurological disorders explains that peaks and droughts in blood sugar levels are often determining factors in people with mood disorders.[k] These mood swings seem to come out of nowhere and the blood sugar imbalances can affect one's ability to handle stressful situations.

The consumption of carbohydrates, especially sugar, releases a chemical hormone called serotonin, which plays an essential role in our mental health and is even used to treat depression. The problem is that that over time we become more immune to the effect of sugar and we need to ingest more of it to get the very same fix. This could explain why the recommended two squares of dark chocolate to cater to our sweet tooth doesn't work for someone accustomed to eating entire chocolate bars in one go.

Willpower

You will often read in fitness magazines and blogs that willpower or a lack of it is one of the main reasons people fail in their dieting endeavours. Willpower has many synonyms including determination, drive, resolve, firmness, single-mindedness, self-discipline, strength, and self-control. In *Willpower: Rediscovering the Greatest Human Strength*, social

[k] 'What is the link between nutrition and depression?' Food for the Brain. 2016

psychologist Roy Baumeister and co-author John Tierney share some useful insights highlighting the role of willpower, its limitations and strategies to strengthen it. One of the most important findings from Baumeister's research is that willpower has limits and gets depleted throughout its use. Indeed, willpower is not only used to resist desires throughout the day (like wanting to stay in bed when it's time to get ready for work), but it is also depleted from decision-making and self-control.

A published survey of 1,328 licensed psychologists found that almost half of them thought that 'understanding and managing the behaviours and emotions related to weight management' were key factors in supporting their clients on their weight loss journey. The participants also found 'emotional eating' to be a significant challenge and obstacle in patients' attempts to lose weight.[1]

One of my clients used to regularly completely cut back on carbs to maintain her ideal weight, like bodybuilders do in their cutting phase. She would keep this diet up for three to four weeks and lose weight. However, she knew that not eating carbs wasn't something she could keep up forever for health reasons so she would slowly *try* (emphasis on try) to reintroduce them. That's what she told herself after every diet

---

[1] Emotions Pose Obstacle to Weight Loss, Psychologists Say | Live Science. 2013

and every time, she would find herself facing completely out of control urges to eat carbohydrates. She would wake up in the middle of the night craving something sweet, 'accidentally' eat an entire baguette in the car on her way back from the bakery or eat her kids' weekly snack supply in half an hour. This would last for weeks and the only way she managed to keep her weight from drastically increasing (she still regained weight) was to run six to eight miles a day. Her mood was all over the place and her family could tell exactly which phase of her dieting cycle she was in by simply noticing how irritable she was. Like most of us, she had willpower but willpower could only take her so far.

Stress eating

There are different types of stress but studies have found that psychological stressors inherent in work and interpersonal relationships lead to an increased consumption of food.[m] This could explain why so many people keep stashes of tasty snacks and treats at their desk.

Researchers have linked the release of stress hormones with overeating and weight gain. Temporary stress has little effect on eating and effects on the body are minimal. But when dealing with prolonged periods of stress the body releases

[m] Mathes, Wendy Foulds, *et al.* 'The Biology of Binge Eating.' 2009

cortisol. Cortisol is a hormone involved in many processes in our body such as controlling blood sugar levels, blood pressure, metabolism, and immune responses. Cortisol also has an impact on our appetite. Our cortisol levels rise as we get stressed but they also drop after the stress is over. If we're dealing with persistent stress, cortisol levels stay elevated and so does our need to eat for comfort.[n]

Have you had enough evidence to convince you that diets don't work? I most certainly have. To cut a long story short and to make it crystal clear, it is not your fault you've been unsuccessful with diets in the past. Like in a poor romantic match, sometimes you have to accept that it's not you, it's them.

---

[n] Publications, Harvard Health. 'Why Stress Causes People to Overeat' 2015

Why your story matters

You may think that the mean comments you make about yourself, both in your head and out loud, don't matter but they do!

Have you ever heard of brainwashing? In this case, the brainwasher is you. In other words, if you tell yourself negative hurtful stories long enough and frequently enough, even if they are not based on evidence, you *will* end up believing them. Not only that, but our mind needs a certain level of congruence to function properly. If you believe that you are unlucky, weak and prone to gain weight because (fill in the blank), you will behave accordingly. It becomes a self-fulfilling prophecy.

Think of your internal narrative and beliefs as a map and your ideal healthy self as the destination. If you are using a map of Los Angeles to visit landmarks in London, you won't find your way around. You can have the best sense of direction in the world, be a positive person, a good person, an intelligent person, but you will still get lost *because* you are using the wrong map.

The first step in getting the right mind map is to change your beliefs. You will be amazed to see how much your story transforms once you identify and let go of your limiting beliefs. Limiting beliefs are assumptions we make about others or ourselves. You may be aware of some but there are a few that just run in the back of your mind without complete awareness, like a computer programme running in the background. Here are a few examples of limiting beliefs: I'm big boned so I will never be slim; I'm too short; I'm too old; exercise is not my friend; I'm too weak; I'm worthless, etc. These limiting beliefs are essentially prejudices we have developed throughout our life, with some potentially inherited from our family, friends, teachers, the media, and so on. It could be as simple as someone calling you 'chubby' when you were a child for you to hold on to that label 20, 30 or even 40 years later.

What do limiting beliefs do? For one thing, they lower our energy by convincing us that we cannot do or have certain things, and by doing so they reduce our abilities to pursue what our heart truly desires, such as having a normal relationship with food, looking good or feeling good.

You may be wondering why we develop them in the first place if they are so detrimental. The answer is simple: by limiting the things we do, think, and feel, limiting beliefs give us a sense of control over our environment. Here's an example: if someone said you were ugly or fat when you were younger, you may lower your standards when it comes to picking your romantic partner because you believe that you are not good enough to attract and keep the kind of person you truly want. This 'default choice' approach is a way to protect you from getting rejected and having yet another reminder that you are not good enough.

Our mindset, as well as our mood on a day-to-day basis, will directly shape the stories we tell ourselves. Freak-outs are also stories. Since I started my business, I've had a few occasional money freak-outs. If you are an entrepreneur or self-employed, you know that cash flow can be unpredictable and for a business, cash is oxygen. Unwavering optimism is often key to an entrepreneur's journey, especially in the early days. I fit the description above on most days but, like everybody, I had my off-days where I indulged in sensationalism.

The story would usually have me running out of money, losing everything, quitting the things I love to do, becoming depressed, and so on... I'm feeling my own energy slump as I write this so I'll spare you additional details. I would usually snap out of it pretty quickly but even a few hours spent thinking this way feels like an eternity. I did lots of work on my self-leadership with my coach Jason Goldberg. With his expert and fun guidance, Jason helped me see that any story can either be empowering or disempowering

A negative disempowering story directs our focus and energy on what will go wrong. This, in turn, makes us less resourceful and creative. It's normal to experience worry in life, no-one is immune to it. The key is to be able to go into 'solution-thinking' mode, focusing on the things that we *do* have control over. To go back to the money freak-out, when I'm thinking about the worst-case scenario I'm directing my attention to a dark future with no solution in sight. When I'm in a positive state (read positive empowering story), I can acknowledge the challenges I'm facing and think creatively of ways to overcome them. When we own our story, when we empower ourselves, we become more resourceful.

The same was true in my recovery from years of disordered eating and depression. I realised that constantly describing myself as a depressed person with an intermittent eating disorder had become an identity. As I said earlier, our mind needs a level of congruence between what we believe and what we do. Thinking of myself as a broken defective person was only fuelling my behaviour. So I stopped. I stopped perceiving myself as a helpless creature. I asked my family to stop treating me like one. If I was having a bad day, I made a conscious effort to refer to it as a bad day as opposed to an expected by-product of depression. I changed my language. I separated myself from the experiences I was having. I learned to stop amalgamating temporary emotions with long term feelings. I stopped believing every one of my thoughts was true. I broke free from the all-or-nothing prison I used to live in. Today, an argument with my husband is just that, an isolated argument and not an irremediable conflict of values. I do not pack my bags and file for divorce. I take some time to think and I leave him space to do the same. Not being able to exercise for a couple of days or being stuck eating sandwiches at work because of a deadline does not mean I am fat, or lazy. It means sometimes things don't go as planned and it's only temporary.

Forgive and let go

There I was, sitting by a beautiful Antalyan beach in Turkey with my then-boyfriend Steve. It was our first holiday together and it felt like a milestone in our relationship; the first holiday usually is. I had just quit my last job and I was very eager to get a break from the busyness and restlessness of my life in London. A French couple was sitting a few metres away, happily chatting. The first thing I did was check out the woman's body. 'She is so lucky,' I thought. 'French women always have the best legs. I wish I had legs like that.'

I've never had nice legs, not even as a child. I discovered I had cellulite on my thighs at the age of nine. Some people like reminiscing about the fast metabolism they had in their teens. You know, when they could eat whatever they wanted without gaining weight. Not me. I don't even have that to remember, I didn't even a get a short stint of body confidence, ever. I'd tried every possible diet; I'd seen a shrink (several shrinks over the years) and I was still fat.

Fat was the reason I was unhappy, fat was what made me moody, fat was what prevented me from fulfilling my potential. Fat was the reason I had so little confidence, so little self-love. Fat was the source of all my worries. It made perfect sense – not really. Deep down I knew it was just a symptom. And because I knew that, I felt guilty. I felt guilty for mistreating the body that had done nothing but patiently put up with my emotional journey. I felt guilty for having an awesome boyfriend, a loving family, supportive friends and still needing food to self-soothe or self-destruct depending on how you want to look at it. I felt guilty for not being happy. Heck, I felt guilty for feeling guilty. I was at my ideal weight at the time, but of course that wasn't good enough because other people were slimmer than me. The French woman had nice legs… I felt guilty about that too. I think you get the picture by now. There was a lot of guilt flying around and pondering on it did nothing to help my situation. I felt like a hamster on a spinning wheel. I didn't come to these realisations on that holiday, but I eventually did get there. I got there by being fed up with being unhappy. I was tired of putting my life on standby. It wasn't fair and the worst part was that it was self-imposed. So I changed my internal narrative and decided to forgive the last person I still hadn't managed to forgive for causing me so much pain. I decided to forgive myself.

You'll never be able to truly move forward and find peace without forgiving yourself for the mistakes you've made in the past, especially when it comes to your body. Yes, you made poor choices, yes you could have done more, yes you could have asked for help sooner. Yes, you could have done many things differently. OK, there is some truth to that, but guess what? That was your best thinking at the time.

You are not perfect nor will anyone ever be. So allow yourself to forgive whatever mistakes you have made in the past, mistakes that have allowed you to learn and grow. Letting go is a key step in this process. Not letting go is the equivalent of nagging your partner on a daily basis for something they did on your first date… years ago. Absurd, right? It took me a while to forgive myself for having been overweight most of my life and for often crossing the line between overeating, bingeing and an eating disorder. I used to wish I was just 'normal' and didn't have to deal with all this 'baggage'. The struggle with food and your body is just one not-so-pleasant chapter of your journey but there is so much more to it. You *can* be happy with yourself, mind and body and a big part of it is through forgiving and letting go.

Why emotional eating messes with your life

If only emotional eating stopped at that: eating. No one talks about the aftermath, the guilt, the disappointment, the self-loathing, and the despair. I remember being incredibly irritable after bingeing episodes. I couldn't look at myself in the mirror because I was so afraid of what I would see. I didn't want to face...me.

One of my dearest friends, Candice, who I met in South Carolina reminded me of other 'odd' things I did at the time which used to leave her completely baffled. Going to the supermarket with me was apparently quite disheartening because I knew the calories for everything and unless she was buying fruit or light/diet versions of food, I would shake my head in disapproval. Candice is naturally slim with a love for good food. She recently reminded me of how I used to cancel our plans to go out at the very last minute because I was no longer in a mood to socialise. Oh, and I felt fat. Candice loved me like a sister and to see me feeling low was both heart-breaking and confusing to her. We'd just spent two hours at the supermarket buying healthy food. Healthy food was *all* I ever bought so how could I possibly feel fat? I'm so grateful to Candice and the host of friends who supported me unconditionally over the years. I know it couldn't have been easy.

I also vividly remember how if I had been overindulging on food for a few days I would refuse to go to the gym until I had undone the damage. 'But why?', I hear you ask, 'It makes no sense! You should go to the gym to cancel it out!' Bear with me here because there were several reasons to this. First, I refused to go to the gym because I couldn't bear the thought of seeing what felt like a mammoth body moving around in a mirror. Second, the thought of being surrounded by slim people who *did* have their life together was so not what I needed. They would judge me because they were so perfect, so disciplined and I was... a mess. An emotional mess. A helpless, fat, emotional mess. The irony of this gym conundrum is that the times I decided to go anyway, despite the mirrors, despite the alleged judgment from other gym-goers, I felt better! I not only felt better there and then but it usually also broke the cycle of self-destruction I was so invested in. Exercise helped me switch off my negative thoughts and shifted my focus on physical exertion, albeit temporarily.

Another side effect of emotional eating, and bingeing in particular, is a difficulty to stay emotionally engaged in relationships. A lot of my clients report a lack of connection with their partners when going through a phase. Not liking how you feel and how you look is not a good combination for a happy relationship. You've heard this before, I'm sure, but the first person you need to fall in love with is yourself. It's really hard to let someone get close to us, either emotionally or intimately, if we can't even stand ourselves.

One of my clients, let's call her Laura, describes it perfectly. Laura was determined to change how she related to food and to work on her self-love. As much as she wanted to, the road to self-love recovery was strewn with curve balls, gremlins and momentary freak-outs. She found herself over-reacting, taking the most mundane comments personally and experiencing extreme mood swings. This isn't easy to witness or cope with for those close to us.

I remember my final attempt at recovery. I had been on that journey at least a 100 times, but I knew that I had finally figured it out. I knew that if I ever wanted to have a shot at being happy, I was going to have to learn to deal with my emotions without any (food) buffers.

Until this realisation, I had considered food to be my nemesis, something of a permanent problem that always required my attention. My fluctuating weight and self-esteem kept me small and invisible. Remember that I lived in the land of 'When I'm perfect, I will be happy'. In my mind, the only thing standing between my dream life and me was the number on the scale. My struggle with food was a part of my identity. It allowed me to bond with countless unhappy people, it protected my feelings (only the bravest would succeed in getting close to me), and it also justified my poor judgement in relationships. If a relationship felt 'too good', I would sabotage it before my partner figured out I wasn't good enough. It justified my alleged lack of professional achievements (heavy hitters aren't usually heavy). In a nutshell, it gave me a perfect excuse to justify my lack of commitment to creating a life I would be happy to live.

As much as we like to tell ourselves that it is just about food and that losing weight will solve *all* our problems, it won't. Figuring out how to navigate the sometimes-complicated web of our emotions will.

Part Two

PRINCIPLES –
HOW TO BEAT EMOTIONAL EATING

What drives emotional eating

Unlike a drug or alcohol addiction, you can't quit using food. You can't check yourself into a food rehab facility where you will sweat yourself out of eating. Food is essential to our survival. Food is readily available. Food tastes good. Food brings people together. Food is love. But like any dysfunctional romance, some of us end up in a love-hate relationship with it. You know the kind, right? You're either crazy in love, happily living in a world of passion or you're looking at the person wondering, 'Why? Why did I end up with someone like this? This is bad.' It *is* bad when a relationship, whether it's a relationship with another human being or food consumes you; when it defines your entire existence. It is *bad* when your happiness is tied to how much you ate or how much you didn't eat. I sometimes used to ask myself, 'How did I end up here?' Not wanting to feel was the answer, that's how I ended up where I was. Eating myself out of life. Shovelling cookies on top my worries, gasping for food whenever something didn't go my way.

You can't look food in the eye and say 'never again', although I have tried. I've tried again and again. I've tried to get food out of my system, both literally and metaphorically. But food and I go way back. We were childhood friends who never let anything interfere with our special bond. Whenever I had a problem, food would pop into my head before I could even process what was happening. If food and I had a relationship status on Facebook, it would be something in between 'In a relationship', 'It's complicated' and 'Waiting for a miracle'. Eating was a reflex, a powerful coping mechanism and the backbone of my resilience.

Resilience is such an interesting concept. No one teaches you how to become resilient and emotionally intelligent growing up. That wasn't part of my upbringing, unless you count 'toughen up kid, that's life' or 'get over yourself' or 'deal with it'. It's only in recent years that we've understood and recognised the importance of Emotional Intelligence or the ability to identify, understand and manage our emotions empathetically. We've also realised that rushing past our problems at 100 miles per hour does not make them go away. So we're learning to slow down because we realise that avoidance isn't the answer to our problems. That's one of the reasons holistic practices such as yoga, meditation and mindfulness continue to gain in popularity. They all help quiet the monkey mind and the restlessness that comes from constantly jumping from past to future, past to future, until exhaustion.

You can't eliminate eating from your life but what you can do is develop an array of tools to help you systematically deal with what's emotionally bothering you. Eating from a large bag of popcorn has some seriously hypnotic qualities. Staring at a screen, hand in bag, hand to mouth, drink, *repeat*. Talk about eating mindlessly. I like to call it a food trance because despite all the knowledge we have about food, nutrition, maintaining a healthy weight and a balanced lifestyle, we perfectly execute our emotional eating routines without any awareness.

What's the alternative? Feeling? As in, *feeling* our emotions? Like many people I work with, I would have done anything rather than feel what was really going on in my life. I had a phase where I decided that if I ate healthy food to distract myself, it didn't count. I sat with bowls of celery, carrots and protein-rich cottage cheese and started my eating ritual, eager to bury my worries under mountains of carrot sticks. Not working... I'll have some grapes... still not working... darn I'm full and I *still* want food!

Before you think I have something against vegetables and healthy food, let me stop you right there. I *love* vegetables, I love my salads, and I happen to love things that are healthy. But healthy food is not what I turned to when navigating boredom, fatigue, stress, fear, loneliness, humiliation, sadness, guilt, anger or hurt. Besides, there *is* such a thing as eating too much healthy food. In the absence of cookies, I would sometimes settle for healthy cereal bars – they worked better than carrots. However, anything beyond two cereal bars in one serving, without genuine hunger, is emotional eating. Emotional eating is typically defined as the tendency to respond to negative emotions by eating, regardless of whether we are hungry or not. The foods we choose when eating emotionally tend to be comfort foods which are calorie-rich foods high in sugar and high in fat, such as chocolate, crisps, pastry, cake, cookies, pizza, and fries. They are known to be highly palatable foods or, in plain English, very tasty.

Emotional eating is one of the main reasons people regain weight after a diet. It makes sense, if you think about it. Most of us now know that regular overeating and being overweight go hand in hand. We can also identify more or less accurately what's good for us (wholefoods, vegetables, etc) and what's not so good (refined sugars, highly processed foods, etc). And yet, we go straight for the biscuits at work, the extra serving(s) of birthday cakes and choose to order dessert even when we feel full.

But why? Is it just plain greed? Are we just talking bad habits here? Can't we use common sense and stop eating when we're full? The answer is yes… and no. Part of the issue stems from deeply ingrained habits (such as eating popcorn at the cinema), and part of it is a genuine craving for food. But as we saw earlier, a craving comes from anticipating the reward we get from a given behaviour and thankfully, that can be tweaked.

In this case, eating initially acts as a distraction. It takes our mind off whatever we would rather not think about, it soothes us, it makes us numb. I had so much self-loathing in my life that the mere thought of being left alone with my undistracted thoughts would send me into panic. What I didn't realise at the time was that the more I used eating as a distraction from what I was feeling, the more automated the response became. Our brain is very efficient and so is our body. If a behaviour is repeated consistently the neural connection becomes stronger. It's like a muscle: the more we use it the stronger it becomes. With emotional eating, we end up associating momentary pleasure, relief, distraction, or comfort with food.[o] The next time we are presented with emotions we would rather not experience, our mind will come up with eating as an obvious solution with proven results. Dr Robert Lustig, Professor at the University of California, explains that foods high in sugar trigger the release of large doses of dopamine in the reward system part of our brain. Dopamine is a neurotransmitter that conveys the feeling of pleasure. The search for more pleasure, consuming more food, results in a change in our dopamine system. He adds that one of the keys to addiction, including food addiction, is that after

---

[o] Adrian Carter *et al.* 'The Neurobiology of "Food Addiction" and Its Implications for Obesity Treatment and Policy.' (2016)

continually stimulating that reward system (all it takes is three weeks), there are fewer dopamine receptors. This in turn means that we need to consume more food to get the same reward. The more sugar we consume, the more sugar we need to get the same fix. [p.]

I noticed this trend with one of my naturally slim friends, let's call her Valerie. Valerie has never dieted in her life. She has never needed to. Her relationship with food has always been a normal one – not too much of it, not too little, she ate what she wanted. We both started working as interns for an NGO on the exact same day. Interning for a good cause is great but one thing that people often forget is how much stress comes from the constant search for the next donation, the next big supporter, the next Government grant. Do-gooders are still human beings and human beings under pressure are not always easy to work with. Sorry if I've ruined anyone's idealised vision of working in the charity sector. It's worth pursuing but it has its own unique set of challenges.

After sharing a teeny office together for eight hours a day and with a great dose of uncertainty as to our future within the company, Valerie and I grew close. We were both passionate about making a difference and, as much as we admired the work that was being done, our own experience within the

[p.] Gunnars, Kris. "How sugar Hijacks your brain and makes you addicted." (2013)

organisation felt rather chaotic. We would start off full of hope and energy in the morning but, as the day went by, boredom and frustration would catch up with us. In an attempt to cheer ourselves up, we decided that a short walk would do us a world of good. What we didn't anticipate was that the short walk would become a ritual that included a daily stop at the nearest kiosk to attend to our 'sweet cravings'. Every day, after eating lunch at our desks reading emails, we would look at the time and then at each other as if to say, 'Ready?' We would happily chat on our way back from the kiosk, thoroughly enjoying our sweet treats. Every day, Monday to Friday, we followed the same routine. That routine was something we looked forward to. In our minds, it was an excuse to go for a walk, a walk we so badly needed to get a respite from our monotonous intern days. Interestingly, telling colleagues at work that we were going for a 'chocolate run' was perfectly acceptable but somehow, we wouldn't have felt comfortable saying that we needed to go for a short walk for the sake of walking. That seemed indulgent. After a few weeks, we eventually realised what was happening – my naturally slim friend picked up on it before I did – and we decided to join a gym where we would attend lunchtime classes.

We started going to an ashtanga yoga class (Ashtanga is a dynamic type of yoga). The class was only 45 minutes long but the teacher was incredibly energetic and obsessed with breaking students' mental barriers about what their bodies were able to do. I had tried yoga back in 2004 in Charleston, South Carolina, and let's just say that it did not go very well. It was a restorative yoga class and at the time I was really big on activities that would torch calories. As you can imagine, based on that criterion, yoga was not my first choice. I feel sorry for the teacher but all I managed to do during that first encounter with yoga was to burst out laughing, snorting occasionally and walking out before the class even finished. I mean, who were these total weirdoes choosing to take time out of their day for this hippie-useless-non-calorie-burning nonsense? Had they not heard of spinning? I know, shocking behaviour!

The experience in London was very different. This yoga teacher was indirectly making me face decade-long limitations I had developed about my body and my abilities; limitations which fed the 'poor me' story I had grown so attached to.

'Poor me, I have no upper body strength, my hips are too wide, my legs are too short.' 'Poor me, I don't have any athletic abilities.' 'Poor me, I work out all the time but never get the body I want.' 'Poor me, I can't control myself around food', so on and so forth. But this teacher wasn't having any of it. He made everyone in the class – regardless of shape, age or athletic ability – execute a rather intimidating-looking yoga transition called chakrasana. Chakrasana looks like a backward roll where you take your legs overhead and push onto the hands, leaving the legs completely relaxed to roll back and end on your knees, or for the more advanced, in a triceps push-up position. When you've executed a transition like that on day one of a yoga class, you feel pretty unstoppable.

This is a very basic example of how my friend and I intuitively decided to change the way we were dealing with stress. A simple shift in our routine – going to the gym instead of going to the kiosk at lunchtime – helped us completely bypass emotional eating at work.

But you don't have to intuitively figure it out because the next section is dedicated to strategies that will help you build up your emotional resilience and bypass emotional eating altogether.

How to manage emotions

What influences our emotions

Our culture places a huge focus on the mind as the main driver for our emotions. What's less common knowledge however is that the body also plays an important role in how we feel. The mind and body connection is not a hoax marketers came up with; it's real. Part of our response to what's happening around us will be physical and another emotional (not necessarily in that order). Imagine if your childhood best friend surprised you with a visit on your birthday. You would see him/her, process what is happening and react. You'll often see people squealing with joy, holding each other tightly or even jumping around with excitement when they haven't seen each other in a long time.

What you think affects how you feel and the way you feel will affect your behaviour. It's called a cybernetic loop. Interestingly, the way we use our body can have a direct impact on how we feel (hello yoga). There is a reason our parents and adults around us used to intuitively encourage us to stand up tall instead of slouching.

Researcher Erik Peper has dedicated a lot of his research to the impact of posture on mood. In one of his studies, he looked at the role posture played in an individual's ability to generate positive or negative thoughts. Peper's work suggests that walking upright increases energy levels and boosts mood, while walking slumped can have the opposite effect and worsen mood for those who were already feeling low.[q]

According to a now very popular TED Talk by Dana Carney based on her research on the benefits of power posing, it appears that open body language and postures in both humans and animals suggest high power whereas closed postures are associated with low power. The research shows that 'adopting high power poses increases explicit and implicit feelings of power and dominance, risk-taking behaviour, action orientation, pain tolerance, and testosterone (the dominance hormone), while reducing stress, anxiety, and cortisol.'[r]

How we use our focus also plays an important part in how we feel. Most of you will have heard: Where the mind goes, energy flows. Whatever the mind focuses on tends to grow. When we focus on a negative scenario, our thoughts tend to amplify the severity of the situation, creating more internal

---

[q] Erik Peper *et al.* 'The Effects of Upright and Slumped Postures on the Recall of Positive and Negative Thoughts.' (2004)
[r] Dana R. Carney *et al.* 'The Benefit of Power Posing Before a High-Stakes Social Evaluation.' (2012)

drama. This is in turn is reflected in how we handle the situation. It's no surprise that so many cultures around the world have idioms to illustrate this idea: to make a mountain out of a molehill, *en faire tout un fromage* (to make a whole cheese out of it) for the French, making a big fuss is another one or, in the Moroccan culture, turning a grain into a dome. We focus on what we *don't* want, we focus on things that are still missing, oblivious to the impact it has on our wellbeing. Our focus determines how we talk to ourselves too; it shapes our personal story. A story can be empowering or disempowering as we've seen in the previous section.

Our focus will also determine the quality of our thoughts and the meaning we give these thoughts. An example that comes to mind is job applications. If I apply for a job and don't get to the final round of interviews, I can draw a number of conclusions:

a. I need to do more mock interviews to boost my confidence

b. They need someone with more experience/a different set of skills

c. I'm not good enough

Each of these thoughts will produce a different emotional outcome. Option *a* is a thought that focuses on a proactive solution, the need to practice more. Option *b* is saying 'oh well, I'm not a good match for this job, let me find something else'. Option *c* gives it a very different meaning. With option *c*, the focus is on rejection. It feels personal because our self-worth was on the line. We made a decision, in some cases unconsciously, that getting the job was a direct reflection of our worthiness.

Decoding emotions

All emotions aren't created equal. Some emotions are quite volatile; they come and go, often unnoticed. Other emotions are much deeper, they can stay with us or even scar us despite our relentless efforts to ignore them. These emotions are part of our intelligence. They let us know when things are 'off', when an issue needs to be addressed, or when we are not in alignment with the beliefs we hold as values.

The most common emotions that can lead to emotional eating are: anxiety, anger, fear, frustration, guilt and sadness.

Anxiety: Anxiety often stems from being exposed to stressful situations and can be characterised by the fear that things will go wrong.

- If your anxiety feels out of control, get professional therapeutic help. There is no shame in seeking the support of a professional to learn tools to help you become more resilient. If you're dealing with mild occasional anxiety, identify the triggers. Consider exercising, deep breathing exercises (readily available online), yoga, meditation, or journaling.

Anger: Anger is usually a sign that our needs haven't been taken into consideration or that our boundaries have been crossed.

- Identify what, specifically, is making you angry. Sometimes we displace our real anger onto trivial things. If the situation involves somebody else and if appropriate, wait until you cool down and discuss how you felt in that situation. Remember that whenever people feel accused or blamed for our unhappiness, they shut down. By focusing on what you feel you are more likely to get into a dialogue that will lead to a positive outcome. If there is nothing you can do to address the cause of your anger, use your self-care tools and support system to help you let go. Exercise is great to let off steam as well as meditation, journaling, reading or using tools like 'The Work' by Byron Katie.

Fear: Fear is one of our most important survival instincts. It's a mechanism that warns us when our safety is threatened or when we are at risk of harm. Fear has evolved over time and now manifests in situations where we are not physically endangered. Public speaking is not a lethal activity and yet it commonly ranks as the number one fear in the world.

- If you feel fear in an environment where you usually feel comfortable (I'm not talking about public speaking or going to an interview), there may be a genuine physical danger and you need to take appropriate action. Any other type of fear can be dealt with in a number of ways. Taking action is a powerful antidote to fear. We try something, and the next time we feel less queasy about trying it again because it didn't kill us the first time. It's natural to feel fear outside of our comfort zone. Every time we take risks, that comfort zone expands and eventually, the previously feared activity is normalised.

Frustration: Frustration can arise in countless situations such as being stuck in traffic, a delay in an order, waiting for a call, or not knowing or understanding what's happening. In other words, we get frustrated when things are not going our way.

- Assess what's actually causing your frustration. Using the traffic example, is it traffic or the fact that you said yes to going somewhere when deep down you didn't want to? If traffic is just a cover up for the deeper frustration, commit to honouring your needs the next time it happens by saying 'no' or 'not right now' to anything that is not serving you. On the other hand, if you're dealing with something that's completely out of your control, let go and shift your focus to something else. Waiting for someone can be an opportunity to sit with your thoughts or catch up on your reading, or if you're stuck in a car, to listen to music.

Guilt: Nobody likes feeling guilty and yet, it is a healthy emotion essential to our wellbeing. Guilt is a way of realising that our behaviour or thoughts are not in alignment with our values and what we stand for in life. It can help us take responsibility for our mistakes. Brené Brown draws an interesting distinction between guilt and shame where the latter manifests as 'the intensely painful feeling or experience of believing that we are flawed and therefore unworthy of love and belonging'. Brené adds that shame can lead to destructive hurtful behaviours that do nothing but exacerbate the problem.[s.]

- Take responsibility for any mistakes you have made and embrace the opportunity to do things differently in the future. We are human and imperfect which makes us bound to mess up sometimes. Ownership is important but so is self-compassion. Once you've taken

---

[s.] Brené Brown, *The Gifts of Imperfection* (2010)

responsibility for what happened and changed whatever is within your power to change, move on.

Sadness: Sadness comes from a sense of loss. We feel sad about death because we miss the people we lost. Moving to a different city can also cause sadness. Sadness is a normal response to an emotional wound and an essential step in the healing process. Trying to suppress an emotion is likely to lead to avoidance strategies such as emotional eating or even drug use eventually resulting in further emotional distress.

- Ask the people you love for support. Realise that as much we would love to be able to fix everything, some things are beyond our control. Give yourself the time you need to grieve the loss and process the hurt you're feeling. The pain will heal and you will get passed it but in the meantime, be kind to yourself.

Whilst feeling your emotions and catering to them is a healthy habit, I would like to draw your attention to the role we play in our emotional wellbeing. One of the most powerful, underused ways to harness our emotions is through our thoughts or, to be more specific, which thoughts we choose to entertain. Yes, there are things way beyond our control that are sad and unfortunate such as illnesses, natural disasters, accidents, deaths and so on. I am not here to tell you that we should become immune to the world around us. What I am interested in, however, is the world we create in our own mind. When I look back at my unhappiest years, the one thing they all have in common is a feeling of powerlessness. I felt at the mercy of my overthinking mind. I then replicated the same powerlessness and lack of emotional agility around food. In my head, food was the culprit failing to understand that my thoughts and the decisions stemming from them were the root cause of my helplessness. My thoughts were all over the place, I could go from feeling on top of the world in the morning to feeling worthless in the evening. Why? Because I chose (yes, it was a choice) to allow my thoughts to dwell on worst-case scenarios, fuelling my internal self-directed Greek tragedy. Master coach Steve Chandler beautifully illustrates this point in his book *Death Wish*: 'When we call a passing thought a "craving" we are dramatizing. Then, after dramatizing a passing thought into a "craving", we notice the sense of urgency it makes us feel.'[t.]

Indeed, a binge starts with a thought. The decision to overeat starts with a thought. The decision to start feeling good also starts with a thought. The thoughts you choose to entertain are always up to you, good or bad, you have the power to turn them into self-fulfilling prophecies.

[t.] Steve Chandler *Death Wish: The Path Through Addiction to a Glorious Life* (2016)

The eating habits to stop emotional eating

The funny thing about emotional eating and weight gain is that it comes hand in hand with denial. I remember trying on my clothes and noticing how tight they were and thinking: I don't get it! I eat healthily, I exercise, how unfair is this? I would go see nutritionists and personal trainers desperate for answers. They would ask me to go over what I ate and everything was... so healthy. Surely, my big bones and allegedly slow metabolism were the problem? Or perhaps I was intolerant to certain foods? I did test after test and... nothing.

It wasn't until I saw a coach a few years ago that I realised that the victim story I was telling myself (I didn't get the same genes as my sister and I get fat just looking at food) was so convincing that it completely clouded my judgment. Talking to her, I realised that my story was so elaborate and convincing that my mind blocked out a lot of the food I ate. My memory deleted all the second servings, snacks before meals, snacks after meals, bags of sweets after lunch. And even when I did eat healthily during the week, I would go completely wild on weekends because I'd been 'so good' and I deserved it. The weekend would start on Friday night and wouldn't end until Sunday evening, by which time I felt absolutely vile and depressed. This was the pattern of my eating in my mid-twenties. The reason I'm telling you this story is so that you can ask yourself and honestly answer the following question: When do you emotionally eat? When do you eat for comfort? When do you overeat? When do you decide to go all out?

The next paragraphs are about identifying patterns and creating alternative strategies to deal with the scenarios where you tend to use food as a distraction or reward.

When?

Many of us eat emotionally as a reaction to stress, sadness, loneliness or even to a feeling of frustration resulting from putting other people's needs before our own. I would like you to take some time to reflect on the different scenarios that you come across in your life. The more specific you are, the better equipped you will be to change your patterns.

One of the triggers I was unaware of for a long time was when things didn't go as planned. A trigger could be a cancelled gym class, not being able to get lunch because of back-to-back meetings, or even getting home very late from work feeling exhausted.

Those triggers are still there. I still don't enjoy last minute cancellations and, living in London, sunny weather is definitely not something I can rely on to uplift me. I have, however, figured out other ways to deal with things that I can't control – I have developed different strategies. Notice that I'm using a plural here because being able to deal with whatever life gives you requires flexibility. As Tony Robbins puts it, '... there will be situations you won't be able to control. Your ability to be flexible in your rules, the meaning you attach to things, and your actions will determine your long-term success or failure.'[u.]

Where?

We sometimes associate food with certain locations. I used to eat popcorn sitting on the far end of my sofa almost every night. When I didn't have popcorn I would feel that something was missing and I would look for a substitute I could snack on while watching TV.

Alternatively, some of the eating my mind used to erase often happened when I was on the go or standing. It's only when I would find the empty wrappers in my bag that I would remember eating a chocolate bar.

[u.] Anthony Robbins, *Giant Steps: Small Changes to Make a Big Difference* (2001)

This is why eating with awareness is so important. First, it helps you enjoy your food more by being present. Second, it helps you realise when you're full. Third, it makes you take responsibility for what you put in your mouth as opposed to going into food amnesia.

One way of helping with the food omissions so many of us are prone to is to pick a specific location to eat. Ideally that would happen at a table with the TV switched off (the TV switched off being the main focus here) when you're home. I would definitely avoid eating in bed as your bedroom would be a space associated with sleep and relaxation.

I understand that the work environment can be a tricky one. The best case scenario would be to eat away from your desk to allow your mind to switch off. If you can't step away from your desk for lunch, turn off your screen while you're eating. If you're hooked to your phone, the same applies. Put your phone face down on the table to avoid seeing notifications.

If you tend to drive a lot and eat on the go, do your best to eat when you stop the car. The same goes with walking, avoid eating while walking, eat before or after you've arrived at your destination. A close friend of mine once told me that she had heard that eating while walking was a great way to burn calories. She found out the hard way that the only thing you get from eating and walking at the same time is digestive discomfort.

The key thing to understand here is that this isn't about making radical changes to your current lifestyle. It's about making small shifts to allow you to give eating the attention it deserves as opposed to letting it happen on autopilot while you're concentrating on other tasks.

Eating formula to never have to diet again

'What can I eat?', 'What should I eat?', 'When should I eat?' and 'How should I eat?' are some of the questions you're probably asking yourself by now. The beauty of the Stuffed approach is that there are no rules when it comes to food because there is no such thing as a one size fits all. Sure, there may be similarities but it is ultimately up to us to find the right formula for our emotional and physical wellbeing. This journey is about learning to reconnect with your body's needs, removing all unnecessary labels and creating a peaceful relationship with food.

Take the example of my older sister Asmaa. For as long as I can remember, Asmaa has always had an amazing figure. I remember her being into sports when she was younger, eating whatever she wanted and never ever worrying about food.

This description still fits her today, more than 20 years later. Having been self-conscious about my weight from a very young age, I used to envy her growing up. To me, she was lucky, blessed with an incredibly fast metabolism and genes I hadn't inherited. What I failed to notice until a few years ago is that my sister didn't use food to cope with negative emotions. To her, food was a source of energy and sensory enjoyment. She never counted calories or tried to cancel out what she ate by exercising or restricting the next day.

Thinking back to my teens, I remember getting so frustrated with her when we went out, because she would rarely finish everything on her plate. The moment she was full she would instantly drop her fork and nonchalantly push the plate away from her. All my mum and I could think was 'What a waste of food!' or 'There's one ravioli left – just eat it!'. Too busy lamenting my slow metabolism, I completely missed the fact that my sister's ability to clearly understand her body's signals was fundamental to her being slim and totally relaxed around food. It's funny how we had similar upbringings and yet completely different outlooks on food. I operated from a place of scarcity (I can't have all the food I want because it will make me fat) while she ate from a place of abundance (there is always more food than I need or want).

If you have a history of dieting or struggling with food, you have probably developed some 'all-or-nothing' ways of thinking. The problem with extremes is that you are either on a diet or you're over-indulging. You're either doing *really* well or you've gone completely off track. You're either obsessing with the food you *can't* have or feeling guilty about the food you *did* have. Neither option is enjoyable, or sustainable for that matter. This can lead to frustration, guilt and self-loathing.

Something else that is common to people longing to lose weight or self-conscious about their appearance is the need for strict deadlines. It may feel like your weight gain happened suddenly, and it could have after being on a strict diet, but it is very unlikely. It takes a while to distort our hunger signals and to continue eating beyond satiety. It also takes time to condition ourselves to make food decisions based on arbitrary guidelines we read on the Internet or in a magazine rather than listening to our body.

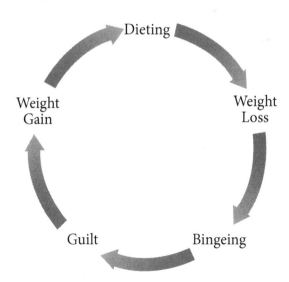

Unless you want to perpetuate this cycle of dieting, you need to completely revamp how you go about the way you eat, the way you think and the way you treat your body.

As counterintuitive as it may sound, I want you to forget about time restrictions. This isn't a temporary fix; you are creating a long-term effortless healthy lifestyle. The initial reconditioning of your mind is the most challenging part. We are all at different stages in our health journey and the length of each phase will depend on what your actual needs are. This is about you and your wellbeing, what other people are doing to undo their holiday eating extravaganza is their problem. Focus on 'doing you' and let them 'do them'.

The less stress, the fewer rules, the fewer negative thoughts, the better the results. I know it might seem difficult at first but I promise you that it will be much more enjoyable than going on a new diet or revisiting an old one which would inevitably send you straight back into the arms of despair. So take a deep breath, slow down and commit to the process, the rest will follow.

We've done quite a bit of work on the beliefs that are holding us back from being our happiest, healthiest selves and you're probably ready to dig into the food section. When it comes to food, it's back to basics. All I want you to remember are these four no-nonsense principles. First, eat when you're hungry. Second, eat what your body wants. Third, eat with total awareness. And last, 'check in' after you eat.

Eat when you're hungry - stop when you're full

- If you had a big breakfast, haven't moved much and genuinely don't feel hungry, don't eat lunch at 12 pm, just because that's when you usually eat. If you have the option to wait, wait!

- Stop when you are full. In order to notice your satiety, you do need to be present. Performing other tasks while eating can distract us from noticing how much food we are ingesting.

There is, however, a caveat with 'eating when you are hungry' which can be controversial. Here it goes: You can eat preventatively in some situations. Let me explain the reasoning behind this statement. If you are going to a meeting from 4 pm to 6 pm and your lunch was at 12 pm, I would recommend taking a snack with you which you can have during the meeting (if appropriate) or straight after the meeting. This is a great way to circumvent the uncontrollable eating that happens when we feel ravenous. The above meeting scenario is obviously an example but the same logic can be applied to any situation (eg. eating something before going to a play which might push your dinner by a few hours, or a long journey home, etc).

Eat what your body wants

- Only eat what you actually want to eat.

- Do not eat something just for the sake of it, because it's available. If you're out and really want pizza, eat pizza – but don't eat three baskets of bread beforehand because they just happen to be there.

- Eat what you want and stop when you're full, no matter how good it is.

When was the last time you ate something you *really* wanted? Until a few years ago, this concept was completely foreign to me. If I'd read the previous sentence, I would roll my eyes and tell you that in the real world people like me end up fat from eating what they want. Yeah, you heard me, *fat*. Eat what I want? Nonsense. Easy to say when you're naturally skinny. The rest of us get fat just looking at food.

But *not* eating what I really wanted didn't work out so great either. I'd been watching what I was eating and denying myself entire food groups since the age of eight and yet the excess weight inevitably found its way back onto my hips and thighs. In my angry, dieting, frustrated state, I believed that if I gave myself permission to eat what I wanted, I would automatically go for junk food because that's what my traitor body would want.

The truth is that while eating an individual chocolate bar tastes amazing and feels pretty good to this day, eating a family size bar doesn't. I don't care what size you are, there is always a point where we feel physical sickness and a decision is made to overlook it.

Let's stay on this honesty train for a bit longer, shall we? Whoever tells you that they can't wait to have a salad for dinner on a cold winter night is potentially hot-blooded or lying to themselves. Our bodies were genetically designed to adapt to different environments and temperatures. We get thirstier when it's hot while in the winter, we tend to crave more carbohydrates which generate heat when metabolised to counteract the effect of the cold.

Leaving all biology aside, I remember how thinking 'I won't have this because it's fattening' used to go down. I would have my Bolognese sauce, without pasta. I would think 'it's totally rich in protein, I'll be fine.' I would be fine, except that at the end of the meal I still wasn't quite full, there was something missing. So I would snack on fruit and nuts. But ten minutes later there was still a little something missing, so I would have more fruit and maybe a bowl of cereal. By the time I went to bed, I would have gulped down over a thousand calories of 'healthy' food. I would feel bloated, and *still* dissatisfied. And this non-stop compulsive eating would all stem from refusing to have a bowl of pasta which would have made me happy and spared me a whole lot of unnecessary eating and digestive discomfort. Moral of the story – have what you want and stop as soon as you're full. The food is not going anywhere, there will always be more food than you want or need.

Here are a few tips to help you choose and make meals that will hit the spot:

- it needs to look good

- it needs to look substantial (no deception)

- all foods are allowed

- forget calories

- learn to differentiate between associations in your mind and what your body needs (a sudden craving for a burger after a McDonald's advert is an association)

Whenever possible, plate your food in a way that makes it look visually appealing. You don't have to be a Michelin Star chef to achieve that. It just has to look good enough to make you want to eat it as opposed to looking like a meal that could showcase in *Les Miserables*. If you are having something ready-made, remove the packaging and place the food on a plate.

This is a big part of making peace with food. It's about learning to enjoy everyday food as opposed to glorifying food that you deem 'naughty', food you binge on or tend to heavily indulge in on 'cheat days'. It's also about ditching the 'boring', 'diet' or 'blah' labels that tend to be associated with healthy food.

Note on hunger by association

Tasty foods activate natural reward pathways in the brain in a similar fashion to drugs.[v] We can easily develop associations between certain foods and specific contexts, say eating chocolate when we are stressed.

Growing up, even as a toddler, I was given sweets as a reward or often as a consolation while my parents were at work. By the time I was seven, the first thing that would come to mind when I was sad or upset was, you've guessed it, sweets. At 20 years old, while my IQ was looking good, my emotional intelligence was at times still that of the little girl who turned to food for comfort. Scientific findings confirm that learned associations act both as a motivational process and result in acquired cravings. The choices we have made and continue to make become conditioned reactions.

---

[v] Philip Werdell *et al.* 'Physical Craving and Food Addiction.' (2009)

Note on deception

You may have read somewhere that using a smaller plate for the same amount of food will trick your brain to think that there is more to eat than there actually is. This visual hack would, in theory, help you feel more satisfied and less likely to look for more food after your meal.

It may work for some, however, in my personal and professional experience, I found that when we go for smaller plates we know exactly what we are doing. We consciously know that we are trying to trick ourselves to eat less and it may cause a rebellious reaction along the lines of 'I know what you're doing, and I'm *still* hungry!' All humour aside, whenever I tried to copy friends at work using teeny tiny plates that could hardly qualify as salad plates I inevitably felt deceived, deprived and… hungry.

This said, if you have ginormous plates that make a two-portion size look like one, I would invite you to downsize. Use common sense on this one and be honest with yourself. Psychological satisfaction is important. If I gave you a salad bowl full of broccoli and green beans, you might be full, but boy would your appetite come back with a vengeance in the evening.

Be present

- Enjoy what you're eating (guilt-free).

- Just eat (no TV, laptops, tablets, phones, etc).

- If you can eat slowly, do so.

- Commit to eating: be totally with it, look at it, taste it, feel it.

This strategy is about breaking the pattern of using food as a way to deal with negative emotions or as a distraction but rather as a way to fuel our body in a loving and enjoyable way.

Check in

- Notice how you feel after eating.

- Notice what your digestion is like.

- Notice how it impacts your energy.

- Notice how it impacts your mood and concentration.

With time and practice, you will become an expert on what foods work best for your body, which food combinations give you the most energy and how much food you need to feel content and comfortable. It's a process, but the outcome will stay with you for life.

Food is fuel, and food is love. Reinvent your relationship with food and your body by adopting a fresh outlook free of prejudice. This shift is key to sustainable physical and emotional wellbeing. If that helps, you can think of your relationship with food (and your body) in the same way you would think of a romantic relationship. In love, it's all about consistency and care.

Imagine if your significant other was nice to you for a couple of days, thoughtful, fun to be around and then, overnight, transformed into an abusive bully only to be back to being nice two days later. Most people would qualify this as an unhealthy relationship and one that nobody would aspire to have. Yet, we create similar dysfunctions in the most important relationship we will ever have, the relationship with ourselves. These dysfunctional behaviours are not only channelled through inner criticism but also through the use of food.

Dealing with cravings and food trances

Yes, initially you may have used food for comfort and to distract you from your emotions, but as time goes on, it becomes more of a habit than a genuine emotional need. And like any habit, if you stop using it, you eventually lose it. Initially, after a diet or periods of restrictions, our body does crave things that we previously denied ourselves. However, even after we've re-gained weight and overindulged on everything we still have urges. Why? Because they have become a conditioned reaction. Whether we like it or not, we are creatures of habits. And in the same way we have wired our brain and body to act on our urges to eat for comfort, we can re-wire our brain by *not acting* on our urges to emotionally eat. We will look at the role of habits and how to create habits in detail in the next section, 'How to break the emotional eating habit'.

In addition to learning how to process and deal with our emotions, there are also practical tools that you can use to help you stop engaging in emotional eating. I divide them into three categories: prevention (before it happens), disruption (stop it after it started) or counteraction (deal with it if it already happened).

Prevention

You know that you are more vulnerable to emotional eating in some situations.

It could be when you're home alone feeling bored. It could be after a night out, after a long day at work, after an argument, when you're worried, hungover or whatever situation you can relate to.

The idea is to come up with alternative coping mechanisms. Instead of staying at home alone bored on a Sunday, you could start a Sunday walk ritual or join a social group or reach out to friends. Make a list of things that usually help you feel good, I have a list of ten activities that never fail to make me feel better. My list includes yoga, dancing, watching my favourite TV shows or calling a friend.

The other side of emotional eating also comes from habit. You know by now that you can have whatever you like when it comes to food, but it's also important to remember that you are still sensitive to hunger/cravings by visual association, as in wanting something just because you've seen it. In order to bypass this 'See food diet' (see it, eat it!) avoid leaving your biscuits on your desk at work. You know you can have biscuits whenever you choose to but there is no need to have daily staring contests with them.

In a nutshell:

- Rehearse alternative scenarios in your head.

- Make a list of plausible things you could do instead.

- Out of sight, out of mind.

Disruption

We all have habits that are essential to our daily life, patterns we don't need to think about consciously. We wake up and brush our teeth, lock our doors, make our way to work etc. By automating our behaviour, we are able to effortlessly execute them and can dedicate energy to issues that do require our problem-solving abilities. But patterns can also be a problem, especially when it comes to eating *because* they run on autopilot.

The good news is that we can interrupt any pattern by doing something unexpected. Have you ever lost your train of thought because your phone suddenly rang or because someone interrupted you? That's what we are going for here.

It's important to interrupt our patterns when we are in an unresourceful state, like when we keep on going over and over the same negative thought.

What are some things that you can do to interrupt emotional eating? You could:

- eat out instead of eating in front of your TV

- cook instead of ordering takeaway

- watch something funny

- write/journal

- jump around in your home for two minutes

- dance or sing your lungs out

- call someone

- do anything that makes you feel good (except for drugs; drugs are a no-no)

Counteraction

Like any other imperfect human being, there will be times you'll make the wrong choices. And that's normal. What matters is how you *choose* to handle them. The first thing I would like you to remember is to keep things in perspective. Your relationship with food didn't happen overnight and it will take time to undo some of your habits, so make sure you take it one step at a time. If you mess up, you mess up. Acknowledge it and remind yourself that Rome wasn't built in a day, it will get better, hang in there. While it may feel like a poor decision has ruined *everything*, it simply isn't true. The second thing I want you to do is to be kind to yourself when it happens and to adopt a soothing approach, the way you would comfort a child who just got hurt. Last, don't just sit there dwelling on what happened! Do something positive to counteract it. Self-loathing always backfires. Trust me, you can't bully yourself into self-love.

Don't:

- Sit on it or lie down straight after for that matter! Overeating usually comes with some digestive discomfort, potentially heartburn.

- Dwell on what happened.

- Beat yourself up (it might make you eat more or carry on the next day).

- Give up, you can always pick yourself up and do better next time.

Do:

- Move your body

- Sit up straight

- Plan your next healthy meal

- Book an exercise class

- Take a shower to relax and metaphorically wash away negative emotions

- Watch an inspiring TED talk

- Call someone you love

- Write about your emotions

- Watch something uplifting

- Do something charitable/make a donation

- Remember you are human and imperfect!

How to break the emotional eating habit

We often mention habits as a luxury – 'I'd love to get in the habit of running', 'I know it's a bad habit', etc. without realising that *we* are habits. Our entire life is made out of habits, tying our shoe laces, using a computer, eating when we're stressed are *all* habits. The processes you have to follow at work are also habits aimed at making sure the work is executed in the same fashion for maximum efficiency and ease. Habits are automated behaviours we developed over time to simplify our life. Can you imagine having to consciously think about everything we do on a daily basis? By automating our basic behaviours, we can dedicate more time to solving more complex problems like writing a business plan or solving a math problem.

Sports coaches place a huge emphasis on their athletes' habits on and off the field. They develop drills, tactics and strategies for different scenarios they continually practice until they no longer need to think to execute them. Military doctors are also trained to develop habits and routines that allow them to think, respond and perform under a great deal of pressure on the battlefield. The entire structure and viability of the military is based on habit formation. Habits are everywhere and the first step in changing them is to become aware of them. Today, we are lucky to have a huge body of scientific work to help us understand the anatomy of habits, their origins and most importantly, how we can change them.

Understanding my own habits was crucial to turning my lifestyle, my work and personal life around. Some habits were easier to change than others but regardless of the level of effort required. We have the power to transform any habit into a pattern that works for us. You have what it takes to replace the habits that have left you disheartened and helpless, time after time. Quick fixes are tempting but they are just that – quick fixes, plasters, makeup, concealer.

The anatomy of habits

There is extensive literature on habits and there is no size fits all when it comes to breaking or creating habits. The most common approach and the one I have experienced the most success with is described in Charles Duhigg's book *The Power of Habit*. Habits are usually broken down into three parts. The first element of a habit is the **Cue** or the trigger, the second part is a **Routine** (actions performed after the cue), and the last part is the **Reward**. This is how any habit is created and learned. Once we learn that the reward comes after executing a pattern, the simple sight of a cue makes us anticipate the reward. It creates a craving.

As a smoker, I acted on a number of cues. If I saw a friend lighting up a cigarette (a cue), I would automatically think that I too wanted a cigarette. The routine consisted of me taking out my own pack of Marlboros and smoking a cigarette while chatting with my friend. The reward in this situation was a hit of nicotine as well as a sense of enjoyment from spending time with my friend. I quit smoking in 2011 after smoking for eight years and what was so interesting about it was that I realised that some people and places triggered my cigarette cravings. Airports are a case in point. As a smoker, coming out of an airport and being able to light up a cigarette was the highlight of my travel (I know, it's sad). Even two years after quitting, every time I travelled I would automatically feel a longing for a cigarette coming out of an airport.

The same went with food in my early twenties. When I was feeling worried or stressed about exams, I would inevitably turn to food for comfort. If a boy didn't call back, I turned to food. What will I do with my life after I graduate? A few cookies will clear my mind.

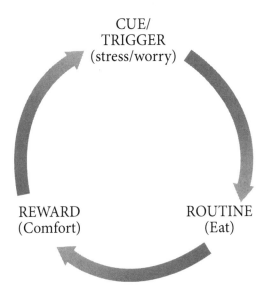

CUE/
TRIGGER
(stress/worry)

REWARD
(Comfort)

ROUTINE
(Eat)

As you can see from the diagram above, the reward comes from performing the routine. For this sequence to become a habit, we need repetition. As we continuously repeat this routine, we start to anticipate the reward that comes from it and that's how we end up with a craving. The repetition is the backbone in creating any habit and in the creation of a craving. You know that eating helps you relax when you're stressed because you've done it hundreds and hundreds of times and this very knowledge will make you anticipate it. It is worth mentioning at this stage that not all cravings are made equal. My friend Charlotte who is a daily runner craves her morning runs and her training sessions at the gym. The craving is the need that drives us to want to engage in a specific behaviour. It's the craving that keeps the habit going without any conscious effort.

One of the reasons so many of us fail when trying to change a deeply ingrained habit is because we try to eliminate the unwanted behaviour (say smoking) without replacing the routine with anything else. Habits have specific functions. If the habit of eating soothes you, soothing being the function or reward, you need to make sure you still get that reward through different means. Remember Cue – Routine – Reward.

One of my college friends Mike who decided to quit smoking started chewing on a straw when he was out drinking. Drinking was his biggest smoking trigger and because he didn't want to let go of his social life which involved going out with friends, he replaced the cigarette breaks that used to punctuate his nights out with chewing the straw in his drink. You might think that's not the most visually pleasing sight but neither is smoking. The cue was still there, out with friends, and so was the reward, having fun on a night out. The only thing that changed was his routine. He might not have done any research on habit loops, but Mike was spot on. Research shows that replacing the 'routine' part of the habit loop is key to eradicating a habit that's not serving you.

In his book *Making Habits, Breaking Habits*, Jeremy Dean explains that trying to get rid of the thought behind a habit makes the thought come back stronger. For people dealing with behavioural problems including drug abuse and overeating, trying to suppress their thoughts makes them experience more negative emotions. Dean suggests thinking of a bad habit you wish to break the way you would think about a river: '... you can't just dam the river because the water will rise up and break through. Instead, you have to encourage the river to take a different course.'[w.]

Creating your Stuffed habits

We try to change a habit by simply removing the routine or trying to remove the trigger hoping that it will last. For a dieter and/or emotional eater, that would mean eliminating any of the foods considered fattening, but what about the cue that triggers them to eat in the first place? Stress, worry, sadness, anger, fear, boredom? Can you remove them from your life for good? What about the reward, the soothing effect that we've learned to get from food? Where would we get that reward?

The triggers will always be around, there is no way of completely getting rid of stress even if you lived in an ashram

---

[w.] Jeremy Dean, *Making Habits, Breaking Habits* (2013)

in India. The key is to change the routine that we use in response to those cues. The routine should also provide a similar reward to that of the old one. But research has shown that having a cue and a reward are not enough. In order for a new habit to last your brain needs to start expecting the reward, it needs to crave it, for the habit loop to stick and run on autopilot. How long does that take? Well, that's a tricky question. The popular answer is 21 days, but research shows that this number will vary widely depending on the habit we are trying to change.

The logic of changing a habit is pretty straightforward but sometimes finding the right alternative can take some trial and error. Finding a new coping mechanism to deal with uncomfortable emotions often requires patience and creativity. I initially tried to talk about my urges with a friend or my mum and that was useful but in my case it wasn't enough. I then noticed that watching a movie with some element of inspiration, movies about athletes in particular overcoming adversity, was a great mood booster for me. But I don't always have two hours to dedicate to a movie and there are only so many movies I can watch that fit this criterion. So while it is a good mood booster, it's not one that I can use daily. Exercise on the other hand ticked and still ticks all my boxes.

I started going to the gym religiously in my mid-twenties but I had zero awareness of the patterns that had been running my life, and my eating behaviours were still all over the place despite my regular gym routine. While most of my friends used to go the gym to help them lose weight, I was genuinely hooked to the high I would feel after a workout session which would give me a priceless hour afterwards of feeling good about myself. We will look into the role of exercise in overcoming emotional eating in the next section. It only lasted an hour initially because I had other habits, like overthinking, that would take over the moment I stepped into my home. After that realisation, I decided to start noticing which thoughts triggered me at home. What were my cues to head straight to the fridge? What happened in my mind to go from, 'I will have one cereal bar as an afternoon snack' to 'I'll have ten of them'? How did I go from having a good day to thinking that I wasn't good enough and burying my sense of unworthiness in food?

The thoughts that made me feel the need to eat could be summarised as: I'm not good enough, I'm fat, I'm ugly, I'm going to fail, I don't know what I'm going do with my life, I'm never going be in a good relationship, X is better than me, I'm a failure. Everyone has his or her own insecurities but they are usually along the lines of 'not being good enough'. What now? To effectively change your existing habits, the following needs to happen:

- Become self-aware: identify the cue/trigger, how you respond to it, and what kind of reward you get

- Change the routine: as we said earlier on, the cue and reward need to stay the same for a habit to change, but the routine needs to be replaced. Find one that gives you a similar boost as food.

- Repeat: repetition is the mother of all learning

The (sweaty) secret weapon: exercise

Whether you are a gym bunny or absolutely allergic to exercise, you need to know that it is scientifically proven that physical movement is key to our emotional wellbeing. Exercising is referred to as the cheapest natural antidepressant available! We often think of the mind and the body as separate but we know both from experience and science that they are closely related. Did you know for instance that the less physically active we are, the less likely we'll be to reach out and touch someone?[x.]

Studies also show that having a regular physical activity relaxes the body and increases our ability to deal with stress. Our mental and physical response to stress is determined by several factors but exercise plays a key role in the management

---

[x.] John Ratey *et al. Spark* (2009)

of emotional and physical feelings of stress by increasing levels of serotonin (used to treat depression) and dopamine known as 'happiness hormones' straight after exercising and in the long term too.

According to Dr John Ratey's research published in his book, the stress that comes from exercise is expected and manageable because we can control its intensity and duration. It shows us that we can manage our stress without using destructive or negative behaviours. In other words, exercise simulates scenarios where we have the ability to go in and out of stress of our own volition. And even more importantly and mind-blowingly, the way exercise impacts how we feel is much more effective than alcohol or food. A study in London showed that as little as ten minutes on a stationary bicycle could lessen alcohol urges in hospitalised patients. Another study showed an hour of yoga boosted the levels of the neurotransmitter GABA by 27%. One of the main functions of the GABA neurotransmitter is the regulation of anxiety. Other studies have found that if people are locked down, either physically or metaphorically, they feel more anxious. Think of the concept of prisons too – we lock people up in confined spaces to punish them for their crimes. So please make sure that you don't consciously or unconsciously keep yourself imprisoned by negative thoughts, exercise sets you in motion both physically and mentally.

If you are new to exercise, my advice would be to find something you enjoy so it doesn't feel like a chore. A dance class, a walk, swimming, badminton, or anything you like. One of the mistakes I often see people making is trying to go from no exercise whatsoever to going all out at the gym. The change is too extreme. Your body will resist the sudden stress you have decided to bestow upon it and the persistent soreness will make it difficult to get past the first three weeks. A lot of my clients start with very short exercise videos from the comfort of their homes. It could be as little as a three-minute workout. You can slowly start increasing the length of the workout as you feel more confident with the exercises. You are better off keeping your workouts short and staying consistent than overdoing it once a week with the risk of injuring yourself. Finding an exercise buddy is also a great way to stay motivated. You are more likely to show up to your evening yoga class if you've agreed to meet a friend there. Having a friend on board or making friends at the gym can make exercise more appealing because it becomes a social activity. Whatever you do, start small and take your time in creating an exercise habit that works for you.

The story of my friend Monette is a great illustration of how exercise can help catalyse change, boost emotional wellbeing and sustain lifestyle changes. I met Monette in 2003, my freshman year in college in South Carolina. Monette is only 5 feet tall but her personality can fill up a room. She was the kind of friend I would call in the middle of the night to pick me up from a college party because I didn't feel safe. No questions asked, she would be there. I loved Monette. I love her. We trusted each other and had heaps of fun together. It is however only now, over ten years later, that we realise that we had something else in common at the time: emotional eating and low self-esteem. Monette kindly agreed to share her story and here it is, in her own words:

Monette's story

Self Confidence isn't something I have always had. I was never the pretty girl, I didn't get asked to any high school dances and I had to ask the guy out for my first date. Middle school and high school kids can be so mean and a chubby girl with frizzy curly hair is a perfect target. This 'teasing' pushed me to develop this hard outer shell that, in order to protect myself, didn't truly let anyone in. This led to many unhealthy relationships. After years of being used and abused by others I developed a new type of coping mechanism. Food became my relationship. Food never let me down, never insulted me, was always there and made me 'feel better'. Something didn't go my way, Ben and Jerry could fix that. Achieved a goal at work, cake! I earned it right, bad day – eat food, good day – eat food. Who needs healthy human relationships when you can have one with food?

Not to say that I was alone during this time, I was married, had five kids, a Bachelor's Degree in Management, I had friends and on paper my life looked amazing. But on the inside I was still that abused woman who hated herself and even though I put on a happy face and spent time with friends and family I was miserable and hated looking in the mirror. I hated the way I looked, I hated the way I felt when I wasn't strong enough to deal with my problems head on and that my only way to deal with them was to eat and shut out everything else around me. This affected every aspect of my life. My marriage, my ability to be a mother, the type of friend I was, everything. My life was falling apart and I was five feet tall and almost 200lbs. My back hurt, I was fatigued, I was depressed, my joints hurt, my menstrual cycle wasn't regular, I had hot flashes, my body was telling me, 'Help, you are destroying me', but my brain was saying, 'Keep eating, food is your only real friend'. I decided I must have a thyroid imbalance, or adrenal issues, or some other hormonal imbalance, it wasn't my fault. So I had blood test after blood test... and nothing. I kept trying to find a reason for my weight gain, but that reason was never 'it is you, it is your choices, it is your habits', I was always looking to blame someone or something else.

Then came the turning point. My husband and I were at a wedding and I love to dance. We spent the whole night on the dance floor. My friend texted me a picture of us with the caption: 'Look how cute you are'. I looked at it and started sobbing. I was so fat. I was so unhappy. So disappointed in myself. I realised it was time. It was time to take ownership and time to turn things around.

I have always been religious and believed in God, and for me it was key to enlist the help of my higher power. For me, this meant kneeling by the side of my bed sobbing. I owned my part in choosing to eat the way I did. I owned my part in letting others control how I felt about myself. I owned my part in blaming all my problems on others. Because in the ownership step I owned that I was not strong enough to do this alone, I knew I needed the right support. I chose my husband and an old friend who was a fitness coach.

The next step was about consistency and goal setting the path to good habits. A goal of 'I will exercise at 1 pm every weekday for 25 minutes' for example. This was mine. Did that mean I had to say no to some lunch dates? Yes. Did that mean when my family was visiting from Chicago I had to stop visiting and exercise? Yes. Did that mean that I had to tell my kids we would play a game after I exercised, but that they were welcome to join me? Yes. Unless it was absolutely unavoidable, I worked out at the same time every day. The longer the stretch of not missing a workout, the higher my confidence and self-esteem climbed.

I was no longer a size 16/18; I was a size 10/12. I felt better, my back didn't hurt, I had more energy and I was happy! I started lifting weights at the gym and I told myself I was working out and that the calories I burned compensated for the calories I was eating. I still had the wrong relationship with food. This is when my husband suggested I train for a bodybuilding show and I liked the idea. I researched coaches in the Kansas City area and decided to team up with a coach, Gary VanRoss. Gary taught me that the first thing I needed to do is realise that food is for fuel. I learned that when I was sad, or emotionally having a hard time I didn't need food, I needed my friends, or I needed my journal. I realised that food tastes even better when you have a healthy relationship with it.

My relationship with food has changed, which has, in turn, changed my relationship with myself. I am a better mother, a better wife, a better friend, a better human being. I no longer have a hole in my heart. My heart is overflowing with confidence, self-love, love from my support group and it now beats healthily. I am so healthy, in fact, that when applying for life insurance I earned the rating of Premium Elite, the best rating you can earn.

Part Three

HOW TO STAY STUFFED –
KEEPING IT TOGETHER

In his book *Emotional First Aid: Healing Rejection, Guilt, Failure and Other Everyday Hurts,* Guy Winch highlights how little prepared we are as adults to deal with psychological and emotional wounds. While most households have a first aid kit in their bathroom cabinet to deal with minor injuries and pains, we have no such thing to treat common everyday life psychological injuries. Winch emphasises the importance of treating these wounds to prevent them from worsening and affecting our mental health.

In the following paragraphs, you will find tips to help you kick-start your emotional self-care routine. Take what resonates with you and leave the rest. Be curious and investigate what helps you feel at your best. One approach might work in a context but not in another, you may find that what used to work for you years ago no longer works. It's all about consciously building up our very own set of 'feel good' tools. Look at emotional self-care like any habit. If you want it to stick, be flexible in your search and consistent in your practice.

How to deal with stress

Stress is so common in modern society that we often underestimate the role it plays in our wellbeing. Stress affects the way we think, feel and behave (remember the cybernetic loop, what you think, affects how you feel and how you feel affects how you behave). The symptoms of stress can be both physical and emotional with signs including irritability, low mood, anxiety, tiredness and aches to only cite a few. We rationally know that if unaddressed, stress can become overwhelming. When we are experiencing physical and psychological symptoms of stress, we automatically go on fight (attack), flight (avoidance) or freeze (inertia) mode. The reactions will vary from person to person but someone who tends to go into fight mode might become more aggressive or irritable. If you have a tendency to go into flight mode, you may choose to avoid the problem in the hope that it will eventually go away.

We are all different when it comes to dealing with stress, but there are ways to feel better which are pretty universal. You may recall from Part Two that emotions act as messengers, neutral messengers. As a part of our emotional intelligence, they highlight the areas of our life we need to pay attention to. If you don't know where to start, try the following:

1. Practise non-confrontation: Don't try to fight what you're feeling; think of the word fight and the negative connotation it brings. The only times two negatives make a positive belong to the remit of physics and mathematics. Have you ever noticed how sometimes being in a bad mood annoys us? Getting annoyed about it only fuels our negative emotions and before we know it, we go from getting annoyed with someone at work to having an awful day.

2. Practise detachment: Like an anthropologist, observe the feelings you are experiencing without trying to judge them. As my coach Jason Goldberg once told me, what if we looked at a stressful day, where we're feeling low, like a cloudy day? Would it make sense to be so attached to the clouds that when the clouds disperse and the sun shines again we would still be thinking about the clouds? Would it make sense to dread the existence of the clouds? Would fearing or hating the cloud prevent their existence? The answer to these questions is, of course, no. You see them for what they are, temporary and out of your control and carry on with your life regardless of their presence. The same goes with stress or any variation of a bad day. There is no need to engage in a power struggle, see it for what it is, distance yourself from the situation and remind yourself that it is temporary.

3. Practise self-care: when we feel stressed or overwhelmed, we tend to put our self-care on hold because we don't have time for exercise or sleep or any other activities that contribute to our wellness. We treat self-care as a luxury. Self-care is always important but in my experience, it is even *more* important when we are navigating challenging times. Catering to our physical and emotional needs helps us counteract the negative effects of stress and prevents us from going into burnout mode.

In the words of William James, '[t]he greatest weapon against stress is the ability to choose one thought over another.'

How to deal with overthinking

The goal of thinking is to look for solutions or lessons to be learned. Overthinking is the act of obsessively going over and over a negative thought or a number of negative thoughts. It's a negative loop where we jump from one negative thing to another, and another, and another until we feel completely overwhelmed.

Dr Susan Nolen-Hoeksema explains that overthinking is to be differentiated from worrying and analytical thinking. Worriers are concerned that bad things may happen in the future, while overthinkers assume that bad things have already happened and start drawing conclusions about their life accordingly. She adds that while negative emotions can give us valuable insights into things we need to pay attention to, overthinking is inevitably tied to low mood and low mood distorts our understanding of reality.[y]

I have more than one example in my own life where a seemingly innocent time for reflection goes rogue. A few years ago, I was giving a talk to Business Administration undergraduates at an American university in Morocco. I put

---

[y] Susan Nolen-Hoeksema *Women Who Think Too Much: How to Break Free of Overthinking and Reclaim Your Life* (2004)

a lot of thought into the preparation of my presentation. I wanted it to be both relevant and engaging to a younger audience and I wanted to make a good impression as it was my first time speaking there. I was brainstorming ideas to encourage students to interact with me and amongst themselves. I had been told that I would have roughly 120 students, how exciting! Hang on, what if no one shows up? These ideas to engage them would be totally pointless. What if the few people who *do* decide to show up don't like me? Some faculty members had also RSVP'd. What if I make a fool of myself? I'm *going* to make a fool of myself! How humiliating! Why did I even sign up for this? Maybe I should just cancel… It's probably a good idea, the last thing I need is for 120 people to realise that I'm not good enough.

This went on and on and on until my sanity kicked back in to finally realise what was happening. This is what Richard Carlson refers to as 'thought attacks' in his book *Slowing Down to the Speed of Life*. He uses a beautiful metaphor about the importance of learning to navigate our thinking the way a captain needs to know how to navigate his ship in any weather conditions. When it comes to our life, he explains, 'most of us resist and struggle with each wave, turning what could be a peaceful ride into difficult, often painful experiences.'[z.]

[z.] Richard Carlson and Joseph Bailey *Slowing down to the Speed of Life* (1998)

Based on your upbringing and personal life experience, you will have developed a number of strategies to deal with the challenges you face in life. Some people deal with setbacks with playfulness and determination, using them as material for anecdotes. These anecdotes put together become the building blocks of their success story. Others will use all their energy to fight back, focused on winning no matter what. A few get completely consumed in the process of overcoming them, plagued by stress and worry. The rest will feel overwhelmed, sometimes helpless, completely at the mercy of adversity. I've dipped in and out of all of these throughout my life, but the feeling of powerlessness is one that used to often prevail.

How to deal with your inner critic

Our inner critic, a close friend of self-doubt, is a voice inside our head that regularly criticises us for what we do, how we do it, what we want to do or who we are even. The inner critic can be omnipresent for some and thus a significant obstacle in our journey to fulfilment. And we think it's normal, unavoidable even. Can you imagine how you would feel if your best friend suddenly started talking to you the way you talk to yourself? *'You look ugly, why are you even bothering with makeup? You look like a cow, an ugly cow! You're going to bomb that interview, who would want to hire you?'* I know it's a preposterous scenario, a friend would never say such horrible things. I agree because your friends love you, and the last thing they would want to do is to bully you. So why is it OK to bully ourselves? Why is it OK to constantly belittle our own achievements? Why is it OK to harshly criticise ourselves when we are most vulnerable? Why is it OK to be mean to ourselves? If someone in my life sounded anything like my inner critic, I would tell them to stuff their opinion where it belongs...diplomatically of course. If they persisted with their tormenting comments, I would completely cut them off. Seriously, I have been bullied so much growing up that I now have a zero tolerance policy for bullying attitudes.

Does this mean you should never criticise anything you do or even aspire to do better? Of course not, wanting to grow and progress is healthy. You are welcome to give yourself constructive feedback and criticism whenever you see fit. Simply note that constructive feedback will have some useful insights that will help you improve whatever you're working on. Inner criticism doesn't. It highlights problems but rarely offers useful solutions. Personal development is about progress, *not* perfection.

The inner critic never shies away from highlighting our insecurities and ultimately validating them by reminding us of all the reasons we aren't good enough. It never runs out of inspiration, creativity or opinions. Your inner critic will always have something to say about you. The key is to learn to make peace with it and weaken the hold it has on you by not paying it as much attention, like a neighbour who endlessly rants about the weather. This non-confrontational approach will give you the space you need to cater to your emotional and physical wellbeing. This will in turn ensure that insecurities and doubts don't turn into self-fulfilling prophecies.

Self-doubt is one of the biggest hindrances to happiness. The more we indulge in self-doubt, the louder it becomes. Self-doubt is also based on beliefs. Remember how we talked about the role of beliefs in shaping our personal story and our identity? Our behaviour will almost systematically be a reflection of the beliefs we have about life and ourselves. In the words of Kelly Lee Phipps, 'If you argue for your limitations you get to keep them'. Self-doubt also fuels fear. When we operate from a place of fear, we move away from our goals instead of moving towards them. If we stay there long enough, we end up looking for ways to escape our suffering. One of the ways of achieving this outcome is, you've guessed it, food. From there, it's a slippery slope. Like any habit, the more we allow our behaviour to be guided by self-doubt, the more automated it becomes. When I felt very insecure, I used to think people at work didn't like me. Because of that belief, I felt self-conscious and took everything personally. When my boss was in a bad mood, it wouldn't even cross my mind that they might be having some difficulties at home or maybe got up on the wrong side of the bed. To me, it was clear evidence of how much they disliked me or how unhappy they were with my work. I felt responsible for other people's mood. My own mood would then be at the mercy of the social weather both at work and at home. If my colleagues were bubbly, I was happy. If people in my team were negative, I would match their mood.

The good news is that you don't need years of therapy to learn how to deal with your inner critic or self-doubt for that matter. You don't need to engage in a power struggle with it either. All you need is a set of simple, effective tools to live your life in alignment with your values and aspiration as opposed to your limiting beliefs.

Let's have a closer look at our inner critic, why does it exist? Consider this for a moment: what if our inner critic was an expression of fear? What if the higher purpose of our inner-critic was ultimately to protect us? What if it was there to protect us from getting hurt by venturing too far out of our comfort zone, like falling in love with someone amazing and getting rejected? Another rejection could leave us sad and lonely, shovelling up ice cream on top of our broken heart and burning shame and who wants that?

Whether it's speaking up at a meeting (what if you make a fool of yourself?), applying for a new job (what if they reject your application, do you really need more disappointment in your life?) or anything else that might disturb your so-called wellbeing, how can we tell the difference between our inner critic and constructive criticism? How do you know if you're constructively evaluating what needs to be improved upon in your life or if you're just feeding your insecurity monsters?

There are a couple of things that differentiate inner criticism from constructive criticism. Notice if the following characteristics apply:

- Mean: It has a mean tone that you wouldn't consider appropriate talking to someone you care about ('Your presentation was awful') or even to a stranger ('What a fat body you have!'). You'll have gathered from the examples that it is prone to berating.

- Exaggerates: It's all or nothing. Making a mistake at work means you'll get fired, a laundry argument with your partner is definitely a sign that you don't share the same relationship values, and missing your train in the morning is yet more evidence of how unlucky you are. Binary thinking or escalating benign disagreements is rarely helpful.

- Compares unrelated experiences: Someone cheated on you when you were 16 would lead you to the conclusion that every other partner you will have will also cheat on you. Or it could be that you won't find a job until you lose weight. I'm still baffled by some of the things I used to tell myself.

- Focuses on problems: Instead of looking for ways to overcome a challenge, your inner critic might choose to stay stuck on why the situation is a challenge to begin with. If you were struggling financially, focusing on the struggle would most definitely not bring you more money, quite the opposite. Constructive criticism and analytical thinking would lead you to brainstorm as

121

many options as possible to get you out of your predicament. The mean voice in your head will also tend to be pessimistic which considerably depletes your ability to be resourceful.

- Unfounded: 'You haven't achieved anything this year!' Yet, when you look at what you've actually done, it simply isn't true. It's not based on evidence.

- Fixed mindset: If things don't come easy to you, it just means you're not good enough. Following that logic, there is no room for growth and learning. This way of thinking makes for a defeatist attitude and, in my opinion, a sad, sad life.

- Unforgiving: It's all about perfection; there is no room for error.

As versatile as our inner critic is, we *can* work around it. With practice, we can get to a place where it becomes muffled and eventually get to a point where it has little power over us. Before we get to the tips on dealing with it, it's really important that you realise that you and your inner critic are *not* one and the same. Your inner critic and self-doubt opinions are just that, opinions. They do not behold sacred truths and the choice to listen to these opinions is always entirely up to you. There are numerous ways to work with your inner critic but let's look at the ones which I have found most effective with my clients and in my own journey.

- Notice it: Become an expert at identifying it. Recognise it straight away by familiarising yourself with the characteristics described earlier. eg. if you're going to be giving a presentation and you're telling yourself that it's going to be an epic fail, you hopefully know that your inner critic is talking

- Distance yourself from it: You are not your thoughts. You are not your inner critic.

- Observe, don't judge: This is an interesting one. The idea is to avoid engaging in a power struggle with our inner critic once we understand that however twisted it may seem, it could actually have a higher positive intent. If you tell yourself mean things all the time it won't hurt as much when you hear it from somebody else.

- Have fun with it: If you think about it, our inner critics are so predictable and cliché that it is laughable. I often call it out by sharing my 'crazy' thoughts with other people. When you say it out loud, it sounds even more absurd. Add a dramatic voice to go with it and it can become hilarious. If you want to hear what mine sounds like, check out my 'Not So Pretty Lil' Lies' video series on my YouTube Channel.

How to put it all together and stay on track

The first thing to remember when you're embarking on this journey is that this isn't a seven-day transformation programme, you don't get fit by going to the gym once a month, you don't learn a language by practising it once a month either. Like anything worth having, revamping the way you feel about food and yourself will take time and dedication. The more consistent you are, the easier it will be. I always tell my clients that it's about the journey as much as the result we're working towards. Every time you notice how you feel and refrain from emotionally eating or overeating is a win. Every time you realise that your inner critic is getting out of control and choose to focus on what is *actually* happening is a win. Every time you feel good is a win. If we don't learn to associate enjoyment with our progress, we lose momentum. If we don't enjoy the journey, we get disheartened and as a result, slip back into unresourceful coping mechanisms like eating.

Here are five tips that will support your transformation:

1. Take it one day at a time

It is great to have a vision and goals for your life. It brings excitement to what we do and helps us be more strategic about our course of action. However, staying laser focused on the daily steps necessary to achieve our goals is paramount. If we've been struggling for some time, the goal can seem so far away and the effort required gargantuan. This can lead us to feel paralysed by the extent of the tasks at hand. To counteract this tendency, there is no better way than taking it one day at a time. Worrying about tomorrow, or our holiday in two months does not bring any answers. Wishing that you could have had it all figured out by now is not helpful either. What is done is done and what matters is that you are here today willing to make the necessary changes to feel good, physically and mentally.

2. Practise consistently

This is one of the keys to successfully transforming your relationship with food. As you repeatedly apply the Stuffed principles in your day to day life, you will notice that you start going on autopilot. You will be completely in tune with what your body needs to be nourished and what self-adjustments you need to make to boost your emotional wellbeing. How long it takes to change or create a new habit varies from individual to individual, but one thing is sure, repetition is key to success.

3. Self-care

Self-care is a necessity, not a luxury. The more you cater to your needs, the better you feel and the more you have to give to people around you. Remember, you can't pour from an empty cup. Self-care will enhance your focus at work, your patience with your loved ones, and your enjoyment of life. I have suggested ways of enhancing our sense of wellbeing throughout the book but you are ultimately the expert on you. Do what works for you.

4. Self-compassion

Feeling good also means having self-compassion. It's having the ability to recognise that weaknesses in certain areas of our life and imperfections are simply a part of being human. When we have compassion for ourselves, we tend to extend the same courtesy to others. It also fosters our sense of resilience by allowing us to recover quicker from rejections and disappointments. Self-compassion allows us to continue feeling good in our skin regardless of the setbacks we may be facing.

5. Gratitude

Acknowledging the good we already have in our life is essential to happiness and growth. Gratitude is a reminder to enjoy what we already have in the present and an excellent antidote against negative thoughts revolving around the future. Gratitude makes us more resilient to adversity and helps bolster a strong positive mindset. Try it on a daily basis, it works!

AFTERWORD

Congratulations on finishing this book and on allowing yourself to be brave enough to believe there might be a new approach to an old problem. I know from experience that grasping something intellectually is a good start, but it's not everything. This book is an invitation to reconnect with your body and see it as an ally as opposed to an inconvenience that can be whipped into shape.

To be clear, this book isn't about losing weight in 30 days or magically becoming so in tune with your body that you will transform your relationship with food in a heartbeat. The transformation will occur and if you wish to lose weight, that will also happen…I dropped four dress sizes over three years because food was no longer a coping mechanism. Many of my clients also lost weight. I don't know where you are in your journey or if you even need to lose weight and quite frankly it doesn't matter. What does matter is that you are no longer at war with food or with yourself. Trust me, you can't bully yourself into self-love. In my case, my shrinking size was just a by-product… of feeling good… good enough.

Feeling good isn't about never feeling low again. It's not about constantly monitoring your food intake. It's not about denying yourself the foods you love, be it chocolate, cake, curries or pizzas. It's about learning to feel without sinking into a dark place every time. It's about learning to feel without feeling less worthy because of it. It's about learning that feeling is normal. Feeling is unavoidable. Feeling is healthy. Feeling is what makes us human; it's what makes us vulnerable; it's what makes us loveable. Feeling Stuffed is about enjoying the journey as much as the destination. It's about learning to love being a work in progress and still knowing that you are enough every step of the way. It's about learning to navigate our emotions and choosing to love. It's about choosing happiness over living on standby. It's about choosing to be happy. It's about choosing to live life fully, right here, right now, no matter how far along you are in your journey. It's about believing you are worthy. And perhaps more importantly, it's about choosing self-love over perfection. And that choice, my dear reader, is always up to you.

Here is to being Stuffed.

FAQs

What if I do need to lose weight?

The Stuffed approach is about finding your own balance. We usually gain weight by consuming more energy than we are expanding. Overeating and binge eating after periods of 'healthy' eating are some of the factors that contribute to gaining weight and staying overweight. By using the principles in this book, you will learn to listen to your internal signals. This means that when you have consumed the fuel your body needs and realise you are full, you will stop eating. Give it a couple of weeks to turn this process into an autopilot routine and watch your excess weight melt away. If you choose to make exercise a regular habit (I highly recommend you do), the transformation will be even more enjoyable to experience both physically and mentally.

What can I eat?

Just like life coaching, adopting the Stuffed approach is all about self-directed learning. This book is here to guide you but you will learn that the expert on all things food and body is actually you. The foods that give me energy and make me feel good may not necessarily be the same for you. Trust your gut and give yourself the time you need to figure out your own perfect food combinations to sustain a strong mind and body. Read Part Two, 'The eating habits to stop emotional eating' for all the details.

Do I need to exercise?

You don't have to, but exercise is truly a game changer both physically and emotionally. It helps kick start the changes you make to your mindset, it boosts motivation and it also helps tone your body. If you need more information, Part Two 'How to break the emotional eating habit' should answer all your questions. Please always check with your doctor before beginning any exercise regimen.

What if I can't afford to go to the gym?

Or 'What if I don't' have time to exercise?' is another question I often get. We make time for what's important in life. There is no need for fancy equipment or two-hour-long exercise sessions to reap the benefits from moving your body. You can walk anywhere and you can run anywhere. There are countless free home workouts available online.

What if I can't control myself?

Trying to control ourselves is what got us here, eating emotionally. One of the main reasons we feel out of control around food is because we have tried to restrictively control our food intake. This is the whole premise of the Stuffed approach. When we've healed our relationship with food and our body, there is no struggle. Food is just food, chocolate is just chocolate, cake is just cake. By reconditioning our thoughts and therefore behaviours, we are able to relax and eating is no longer a way of coping with emotions or a source of anxiety in and of itself.

What if I'm travelling?

The same principles apply when you're travelling. This being said, you may well be in tune with your body but find you only have limited options. Do the best you can with what's available. You may even find that you indulge a bit more than you would while you're home but that's absolutely fine. You may even find that you've have gained a little bit of weight (your clothes can tell you that without needing a scale) and that's fine too.

A client of mine went to Italy for a couple of days and her diet while there consisted of wine, cheese, pasta and more wine. She was concerned that she was gaining weight and already anticipating how she would have to undo the damage when she came back. After a brief phone intervention, she relaxed and while she was still indulging in wine, cheese, and pasta, she decided to actually enjoy it as opposed to feeling guilty about it or trying to have as much of it as possible because of the looming diet that used to always await her after a holiday. She enjoyed the food, listened to her body and had fun. By the time she went back to London, she was looking forward to vegetable rich meals, fruit and CrossFit training sessions in the morning. She was craving her normal lifestyle because it felt good, because she designed it to suit her needs.

What about cheat meals/cheat days?

There is no need for cheat meals or cheat days when you are Stuffed because you don't have to wait for a particular day of the week to have what you want. You don't need to go overboard either because you know you can have what you want any time. Consider anything you want to have, that you wouldn't necessarily fancy on a daily basis, as a *treat* rather than a cheat snack/meal/day/hour… The idea of a cheat meal is based on the assumption that you are only allowed to have some food for a limited period of time and that, my friends, is how we become obsessed with food and start bingeing. Food is there, you can have as little or as much as you want as long as you are listening to your body and following the simple principles you've learned in this book. If you fancy cake for breakfast on holiday, have it! If everyone is having ice cream but you want a green smoothie, that's cool too. It's called living life and eating on your terms!

How do I deal with people I share my life with who don't eat the way I do?

This isn't a diet and it should therefore be really easy to eat around other people as you can still eat what you want to eat. Once you re-establish that mind-body connection, you may find that you are naturally attracted to more wholesome foods or that you eat exactly what you used to but just less of it because you now know when you're full. Neither one of these options requires self-control or restriction, just self-awareness. Am I full? How do I feel after eating a particular type of food? What do I actually want to eat? What does my body need?

Think of it this way, if your significant other *really* liked cream cheese and marmite and you *really* disliked them, would that be a problem? My guess is no; you may not love these foods but they do. Would you try to convert them to *not* liking these foods? 'Look, we really need to have a talk about cream cheese, I don't think you should carry on eating it.' Of course not! It's only when we talk about diets and particular nutrition plans that are restrictive by nature that we start seeing conflicting agendas. What you eat and how much of it you eat will be very personal to you. And just like you probably wouldn't feel pressured to like cream cheese, there is no need to feel guilty about eating what you want to eat, even if it's different to what others are eating around you. The key is to not make a fuss about it and resist the temptation to preach *your* way of relating to food.

How long will it take?

It all depends on where you are starting. Typically, it takes a few weeks to really grasp the logic of this approach (your inner critic will be battling you on that one) and another few weeks of committed practice. Mindset and self-awareness are fantastic starting points, but taking consistent action is key to cement it all and to start noticing changes.

You can do it at your own pace but what I will say is that if you don't take consistent action straight away, really committing to the process, you will lose the momentum and this book will be just another thing you tried.

Can I weigh myself?

You are free to do so but I always recommend using different means to check in or measure your progress that are more relevant. I know how hard it is to let go of the thought that your weight is important. The number on the scale can fluctuate from one day to another and weighing less does not always mean that we are fitter or healthier. Muscle weighs more than fat, foods high in salt cause water retention, hormonal changes and many more factors can influence what you read on the scale. It's simply not accurate. If you are healthy, if you love how you look and feel good in your body, why allow an arbitrary number to define your happiness?

Plus let's be honest here, the number you see on the scale will *always* result in a reaction. You can tell yourself that it keeps you motivated but you and I know that while this may be true *sometimes*, it is more often than not disheartening.

If weighing yourself causes you stress and anxiety, *ditch your scale*. Hide it, give it to a charity shop or just get rid of it. There are so many other ways to measure your progress and wellbeing. For one, look in the mirror, notice how your clothes fit, your energy levels, your mood and your strength.

What about juicing and other detoxes?

I don't want to generalise here, but my guess is that if you have picked up this book, you (or someone you know) have had your fair share of challenges in the food/body arena. Some juicing and detoxes have health benefits but a lot of them are just other marketing attempts to re-brand and sell extreme diets.

I have worked really hard to get to a place where I'm at peace with myself and my body and I know that trying anything that restricts food or that even remotely reminds me of a diet can trigger old dysfunctional eating patterns which usually result in binges. My advice would be to avoid any juicing or detoxes unless it is something prescribed by your doctor. For more information on why dieting and restricting foods doesn't work go back to Part 1, 'Why you can't stick to a diet'.

BIBLIOGRAPHY

Brown, Brené C. *The Gifts of Imperfection: Let Go of Who You Think You're Supposed to Be and Embrace Who You Are.* Philadelphia, PA, United States: Hazelden Information & Educational Services, 2010. Print.

Baumeister, Roy F., and John Tierney. Willpower: Rediscovering the Greatest Human Strength. New York: Penguin Putnam, 2011. Print.

Chandler, Steve. *Death Wish: The Path Through Addiction to a Glorious Life.* United States: Maurice Bassett, 2016. Print.

Robbins, Anthony. *Giant Steps: Small Changes to Make a Big Difference.* New York: Pocket Books, 2001. Print.

Winch, Guy. *Emotional First Aid: Practical Strategies for Treating Failure, Rejection, Guilt, and Other Everyday Psychological Injuries.* New York, NY, United States: Hudson Street Press (an imprint of Penguin Group (USA) Inc), 2013. Print.

Nolen-Hoeksema, *Susan. Women Who Think Too Much: How to Break Free of Overthinking and Reclaim Your Life.* 2nd ed. London: Piatkus Books, 2004. Print.

Hansen, Kathryn. *Brain Over Binge: Why I Was Bulimic, Why Conventional Therapy Didn'T Work, and How I Recovered For Good.* United States: Camellia Publishing, 2011. Print.

Ratey, John J, and Eric Hagerman. *Spark.* London: Quercus Publishing Plc, 2009. Print.

Duhigg, Charles. *The Power of Habit: Why We Do What We Do in Life and Business.* New York: Random House Publishing Group, 2012. Print.

Aamodt, Sandra. *Why Diets Make Us Fat: The Unintended Consequences of Our Obsession with Weight Loss.* United States: Current, 2016. Print.

Dean, Jeremy. *Making Habits, Breaking Habits.* Great Britain: Oneworld Publications, 2013. Print.

Carlson, Richard, and Joseph Bailey. *Slowing down to the Speed of Life: How to Create a More Peaceful, Simpler Life from the Inside out.* San Francisco: HarperSanFrancisco, 1998. Print.

Kalm, Leah M., and Semba, Richard D. 'They Starved So That Others Be Better Fed: Remembering Ancel Keys and the Minnesota Experiment.' *The Journal of Nutrition* 135.6 (2005): 1347. Web.

Harkness, Jon M., and Todd Tucker. 'The Great Starvation Experiment: Ancel Keys and the Men Who Starved for Science.' *The Journal of American History* 96.1 (2009): 278. Web.

Gunnars, Kris. 'How sugar Hijacks your brain and makes you addicted.' Health. Authority Nutrition, 26 Jan. 2013. Web. 3 Nov. 2016.

Avena, Nicole M., Rada, Pedro, and Hoebel, Bartley G. 'Evidence for Sugar Addiction: Behavioral and Neurochemical Effects of Intermittent, Excessive Sugar Intake.' *Neuroscience & Biobehavioral Reviews* 32.1 (2008): 20-39. Web.

Carter, Adrian, *et al.* 'The Neurobiology of "Food Addiction" and Its Implications for Obesity Treatment and Policy.' *Annual Review of Nutrition* 36.1 (2016): 105-128. Web.

Mathes, Wendy Foulds, Kimberly A. Brownley, Xiaofei Mo, and Cynthia M. Bulik. 'The biology of binge eating.' *Appetite* 52.3 (2009): 545-553.

White, Marney A., *et al.* "Development and Validation of the Food-Craving Inventory." *Obesity Research* 10.2 (2002): 107–114. Web.

Werdell, Philip et al. 'Physical Craving and Food Addiction' The Food Addiction Institute (2009). A Scientific Review Paper. Web

Harvard Health Publications. Why stress causes people to overeat – Harvard health. 20 May 2015. Web. 2 Nov. 2016.

Fedoroff, Ingrid, Janet Polivy, and C Peter Herman. 'The specificity of restrained versus unrestrained eaters' responses to food cues: general desire to eat, or craving for the cued food?' *Appetite* 41.1 (2003): 7-13. Web.

Sánchez-Villegas, Almudena, *et al.* 'Fast-Food and Commercial Baked Goods Consumption and the Risk of Depression.' Public Health Nutrition 15.03 (2011): 424–432. Web.

Wilson, Vietta, and Peper, Erik. 'The Effects of Upright and Slumped Postures on the Recall of Positive and Negative Thoughts.' *Applied Psychophysiology and Biofeedback* 29.3 (2004): 189-195. Web.

Pelchat, Marcia Levin, and Susan Schaefer. 'Dietary Monotony and Food Cravings in Young and Elderly Adults.' *Physiology & Behavior* 68.3 (2000): 353–359. Web.

McCabe, Randi E., 'Exposing the diet myth: diets make you eat less', National Eating Disorder Information Centre (1999). Web.

Cuddy, Amy J.C., Caroline A. Wilmuth, and Dana R. Carney. 'The Benefit of Power Posing Before a High-Stakes Social Evaluation.' *Harvard Business School Working Paper*, No.13-027 (2012). Web.

Nauert, Rick. *Poor eating behaviors can worsen mood | Psych central news. Psych Central News*, 18 Mar. 2013. Web. 28 Oct. 2016.

Swayne, Matthew. *Unhealthy eating can make a bad mood worse | Penn state university.* 28 Oct. 2016. Web. 28 Oct. 2016.

Lallanilla, Marc. How Junk Food Makes a Bad Mood Worse | Live Science. 18 Mar. 2013. Web. 28 Oct. 2016.

Emotions Pose Obstacle to Weight Loss, Psychologists Say | Live Science. 18 Mar. 2013. Web. 28 Oct. 2016.

'What is the link between nutrition and depression?' *Food for the Brain*. 2016. Web. 01 Nov. 2016.

ACKNOWLEDGEMENTS

To my mum and dad, I am so grateful for all you've done and continue to do to support me. I wouldn't be so dedicated to helping others if it weren't for you leading by example. I love you both so much.

To Steve, my husband and anchor. Thank you for your unwavering love and belief in me. Thank you for teaching me how to be more playful about the little things in life. You are the embodiment of fun and light-heartedness. I love you!

To Asmaa, my sister, number one fan, best friend, and role model. I wouldn't be who I am today if it weren't for you. Thank you for all that you are and for who you inspire me to be.

To Narmine, my big sister, for showing me how to live my life for me, regardless of what people think. You will never cease to surprise me!

To Jason Goldberg, for teaching me how to unleash my creativity with fun and authenticity. Thank you for your coaching, mentoring and friendship, you have completely shifted the way I experience the world and I can never thank you enough for that.

To Michael Serwa, friend and coach, for welcoming into the world of personal development with open arms, telling me exactly what I needed to hear and for relentlessly encouraging me to raise my standards.

To Duda, my muse. I love you dearly and I am so grateful to have you in my life.

To my coaching tribe, Tomas, Tadj, and Raghav. I couldn't wish for a better gang; I feel invincible around you guys!

To Jane A. Zazzaro, Nina Papadopoulos, Amani Zarroug, and Diana Battle for helping feel 'Stuffed'.

Last but not least, to my amazing clients, for trusting me to be a part of your journey and for inspiring me to always play a bigger game.

THE AUTHOR

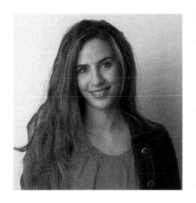 Fadela is a Life Coach and speaker specialising in helping busy successful entrepreneurs who thrive in business but lack in their personal life and wellbeing. She helps her clients uncomplicate their emotions so that they can focus on their purpose.

Trained in Coaching and Neuro Linguistic Programming, Fadela also holds a Masters in Conflict, Security and Development from King's College London and Bachelor degrees in Economics and Spanish from the College of Charleston (US). Using her international experience working in the private sector and charity sector, Fadela creates multidisciplinary and culturally-aware solutions for her clients all over the world. Fadela's motto is 'feel good, do good'.

She is also the founder of Prayanas, a company specialising in leadership, learning and development. Prayanas delivers a range of tailored training and coaching programmes for global organisations, businesses, universities and not-for-profits.

To find out more about Fadela Hilali, visit:
www.prayanas.com

You can also connect with her on social media:
Twitter: www.twitter.com/fadelahilali
Facebook: www.facebook.com/FadelaWellbeing
Linkedin: www.linkedin.com/in/FadelaHilali
YouTube: www.youtube.com/fadelahilali

33247611R00090

Printed in Great Britain
by Amazon